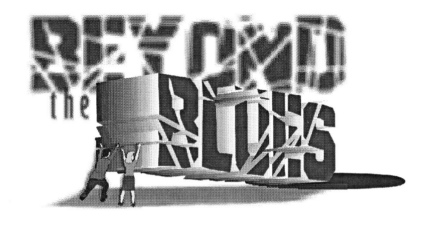

Treating Depression One Day at a Time

W0008249

Edward F. Haas

Copyright © 2000 by Edward F. Haas

ISBN 0-7414-0086-3

Published by:

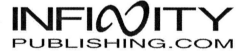

PUBLISHING.COM

Infinity Publishing.com
519 West Lancaster Avenue
Haverford, PA 19041-1413
Info@buybooksontheweb.com
www.buybooksontheweb.com
Toll-free (877) BUY BOOK
Local Phone (610) 520-2500
Fax (610) 519-0261

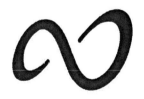

Printed in the United States of America

Printed on Recycled Paper

Published October-2000

Dedicated to the loving memory of my friend
Brian S. Hamaker 1954-1997

I will always regret that I didn't do more to help.

Acknowledgments

The path in which I have traveled to bring me to the point of writing an acknowledgment page for a daily meditation book designed for people who suffer from clinical depression, is absolutely remarkable in my estimation. I have concluded that every single moment of my life, every happening, every word spoken or heard, positively everything that has occurred in my life prior to this moment is responsible for it. The support I have received during this journey has been truly wonderful.

First, to my wife Cina, and my sons, Aaron and Ryan...I am so blessed to have each of you in my life today. To my editing crew...Holly Newstein, Jan Cremer, John Torbet, and Susan Burtnett. Without your encouragement and honest appraisal, this book would be filled with many embarrassing mistakes. Thank you. To Brian Halstead and Jeff Ross...your friendship and support have helped to keep me alive long enough to write a book. Absolutely amazing!

Also, I want to thank Holly, Brian, Jeff, and John for their written contributions. During my "blocks" your efforts inspired me to write on.

And finally, to that Great Spirit in the sky...Peace be still.

January1

Thought for the day
It has long since come to my attention that people of accomplishment rarely sat back and let things happen to them. They went out and happened to things.

Elinor Smith

Meditation
As another year passes, take a moment to consider where you were and what you were doing one year ago. Are you better off today...or are you in a lot of pain because of some new crisis that has crept into your life? If so, can you not find solace in the idea that you do not have to needlessly suffer alone...that if you choose, you may reach out for comfort and support from another person who also suffers from depression. Or maybe you're just beginning your recovery process, scared to death, not believing for one minute that you will ever know serenity and peace in your life again. My friend I say to you, "carry on". Don't give up on yourself. You are alive today for a reason, and although I can't tell you exactly what that reason may be...I can tell you with absolute certainty that it is *not* to kill yourself. So don't just sit back and wait for something better to happen in your life. Get up and be on your way to the road of recovery and a happier destiny.

Prayer
God, I pray that you will continue to work your miracles within the community of depression sufferers. In large cities, people that are afflicted with this disease meet regularly to support one another. I ask that you will help this movement solidify and spread so that all that are lost in the darkness of despair may soon know peace. Amen

January 2

Thought for the day
Faith moves mountains, but you have to keep pushing while you are praying.

Mason Cooley

Meditation
God knows we have done some praying! Many of us have prayed to die. Some of us have attempted suicide and failed. Others will not make the attempt to take their own lives, but nevertheless, will still not put up much of a fight if some external condition or event threatened them. What a horrible way we have lived! Only those of us who have been to the black hole know this insanity. God does not want us to travel this road alone. We must remember to ask for help. That is our biggest push against the mountain.

Prayer
God, please give me the courage and strength to ask for help when I recognize a bout of depression setting in. Please help me to also be available for my fellow sufferers when they reach out for help. Amen

January 3

Thought for the day
Do what you can, with what you have, where you are.

Theodore Roosevelt

Meditation
Part of my treatment of depression is accepting that some days I am not going to feel very well at all. Some days, the best that I will be able to hope for is to just get by. I have to accept that there will be days that all I can look forward to is when the darkness will lift. My experiences in recovery tell me that the day will eventually come. I must accept that I am going to exhibit the symptoms of my illness. By accepting the fact that I suffer from this illness called depression, I can better live with it.

Prayer
God, help me to accept the reality of my condition. Help me to remember that I will have periodic bouts with depression. Help me to do what I can, with what I have, wherever I am. Amen

January 4

Thought for the day
He has half the deed done who has made a beginning.

Horace

Meditation
I suffer from cyclic depression. I always know when I am slipping into the black hole. It never happens suddenly for me. It is always a slow decline over a period of approximately two weeks. Each day that I slip a little deeper, I convince myself that my feelings must be the result of some external condition. I find myself scrambling to find some person or situation to put blame on. If I cannot find anything current, I will dredge up the past. I must find a reason for my feelings of worthlessness or else I will know that I am just plain nuts! Usually, it doesn't add up. In my mind I scramble some more. By now my family is beginning to look at me a little funny. At last, it happens. I realize that my feelings of worthlessness are nothing more than an episode with depression. I pick up the phone and call for help. Sometimes I call my doctor. Other times I call a friend. The result is always the same. At the moment that I "make the beginning" and ask for help, I experience some immediate relief.

Prayer
God, help me to always make the beginning, and ask for help. Help me quickly realize that when I begin to experience those feelings of worthlessness, I am exhibiting the symptoms of depression. Thank you for the recovering people who have been there to answer my calls for help. Amen

January 5

Thought for the day
When spider webs unite, they can tie up a lion.

Ethiopian proverb

Meditation
How strong is the fellowship between fellow sufferers? If it were not for my "web" of relationships with other people who also suffer from depression, there is a very good chance that I would no longer be alive. What a blessing I have found. It makes my life so much more enjoyable knowing that at any time I can call upon one of the many contacts that I have, to talk about my depression. It is also very rewarding to be able to help a fellow sufferer through a difficult time. For people like us, to isolate is to die. We must reach out to others for help. When we unite, we have the strength to "tie up our lion".

Prayer
God, please give me the courage to reach out to the "web" of fellow sufferers. Help me to remember that this illness wants to isolate and then kill me. I cannot fight depression on my own. I must have the support of others who have been through the " valley of darkness". Please light my way. Amen

January 6

Thought for the day
Let me tell you the secret that has led me to my goal. My strength lies solely in my tenacity.

Louis Pasteur

Meditation
Do not give into your self-defeating thoughts. Fight the good fight. The reason I am still alive today is because, after many failed attempts at recovery from alcoholism, cocaine addiction, and depression, I continued to ask for help. It was during my most hopeless stages that I found my greatest strengths. Be tenacious! Do not believe the lies that your illness is telling you. You do not have to live in a dark hole of despair. Reach out and find the healing that you need. Be willing to reach as often and as far as it takes for you to find your solution!

Prayer
God, please grant me the willingness to fight the good fight. Help me remember that hundreds of thousands of fellow sufferers have found the healing which they so desperately sought...healing that is also available to me. Amen

January 7

Thought for the day
Every calling is great when greatly pursued.

Oliver Wendell Holmes, Jr.

Meditation
I believe it is my responsibility to help others who suffer from depression. Just as I make myself available to alcoholics and drug addicts, I also have to be available to any person who suffers from this disease. Helping others in their recovery process has turned out to be the most effective way for me to help myself. I believe it is God's will for me. It does not require a great deal of effort either. I simply make certain I am present when I can be. I am quick to share my personal testimony with others if they are willing to listen. I am liberal with my phone number. I encourage anyone who needs to call me, to do so. My blessing is that I found this kind of support when I started out on my road to recovery.

Prayer
God, please grant me the strength to answer your call. Help me remember how you blessed me by putting loving, caring people into my life. Encourage me to provide time in my life to help others. Thank you for the blessings that helping others has and will continue to bring me. Amen

January 8

Thought for the day
The reward of a thing well done, is to have done it.
Ralph Waldo Emerson

Meditation
The reward of reaching out from the darkness is life. It is the reaching itself that becomes our "thing well done". Treating depression requires effort. Raising our bottom out of the darkness and stabilizing requires vigilance. Just as the alcoholic is usually the last to know there is a problem, so it is for us who suffer from depression. To treat our depression is a "thing well done". To ignore it, with the hope it will go away...is mental, spiritual, and perhaps physical death.

Prayer
God thank you for the support you have made available to me. Thank you for the strength to reach out for help. Thank you for reminding me that I am not alone with this illness. Thank you for revealing to me that by reaching out for help, and by treating my depression, I have done well. Amen

January 9

Thought for the day
A walking shadow, a poor player, that struts and frets his
hour upon the stage and then is heard no more.

Shakespeare, 'Macbeth'

Meditation
A walking shadow, a poor player... When I am suffering,
that is how I feel. But that is not what I am! I must always
remember that I am not depression. I only suffer from it.
When I am in the black hole, I strut and fret. If I do not get
help, I suffer needlessly. Some of us die and are " heard no
more". I must maintain constant vigilance to identify the
symptoms as they begin. I must recognize them before I am
in too deep. I know that at the deepest depths of despair it is
so difficult to reach out for help.

Prayer
God, please grant me the wisdom to separate myself from
this illness. Help me believe that I am not a "walking
shadow". In my darkest, most difficult moments, please
guide me toward your saving grace. Help me find your light.
Amen

January 10

Thought for the day
Action precedes motivation.

Unknown

Meditation
It is the Catch-22 of depression. Taking action can begin to relieve some of the pain. Doing *something* can improve my mood. But the paradox here is that a symptom of depression is the inability to start anything. How many hours have I spent in bed, feeling the pain, unable to begin even the smallest activity? How much time have I wasted, waiting for the motivation to move? The challenge is to take action despite my unwillingness to do so. And this start, however small, can be the turning point in a depressive episode. Indeed, it may even save my life. It can be as simple as a phone call – to my doctor, therapist, or a fellow sufferer, who can understand what I am going through.

Prayer
Lord, I pray that I may be able to take action when I need to. Give me the strength to begin when I am without motivation. Amen.

January 11

Thought for the day
Noble deeds and hot baths are the best cures for depression.

Dodie Smith

Meditation
Not our type of depression! I have often wished I could find another word for the type of depression I suffer from. It is so frustrating trying to explain clinical depression to someone who does not understand. We usually get responses such as…" What do you have to feel so bad about?" Or…"Why don't you just be grateful for what you have?" And, "Stop feeling so sorry for yourself!" I used to walk away from these conversations feeling very frustrated. I have since learned that my illness is real. I have also learned that I do not have to make a single person understand it. What is important today is that I take personal responsibility for my own recovery and treat my depression on a daily basis. That treatment may include medications. It may include a support group. It may also include an occasional hot bath!

Prayer
God, please grant me the knowledge to not feed into the lies and ignorance that surround clinical depression. Help me remember that I am not an ungrateful, selfish person. Please remind me that I am just a sick person trying to get well. Amen

January 12

Thought for the day
When written in Chinese, the word crisis is composed of two characters. One represents danger and the other represents opportunity.

John F. Kennedy

Meditation
When I was suffering from depression...but didn't realize that I was exhibiting the symptoms of an illness, I was in a crisis. I was caught up in a vicious cycle of alcohol, cocaine, and depression. Every time I would attempt to get "clean" from the alcohol and cocaine, I would slip into a major depression. The only solution that I knew of to deal with the depression was to self-medicate with more alcohol and cocaine. This of course kept me stuck in the sick cycle. I finally reached a hopeless point where suicide seemed like the only true solution to my problem. But for the grace of God, a person was put into my life that pointed me in the right direction. I started treating my depression, alcoholism, and chemical dependency, all at once. Through my crisis the most wonderful opportunities have been bestowed upon me. I am clean and sober! I have wonderful support from my family and friends. I share my experience, strength, and hope with others. What a wonderful gift I have been blessed with.

Prayer
God, please help me see your good in all things. Remind me that you did not save me from drowning just to smash me against the rocks of the shore. Amen

January 13

Thought for the day
Everything comes to him who hustles while he waits.

Thomas A. Edison

Meditation
When I find myself exhibiting the symptoms of depression, I need to hustle. I need to reach out for help with a sense of urgency. The deeper I allow myself to sink, the harder it becomes to get out of the black hole. Sometimes I make a series of calls and then wait for callbacks. If I need to see my doctor, rarely will he be able to see me that same day. I have to continue with all my efforts until my appointment. Sometimes, I have to force myself not to isolate from my family and friends. Maybe I'll try to get together with some people who make me laugh…people who know what I am going through. We have all learned that laughter can do wonders to take the edge off. The worst thing I can do is allow myself to be consumed with depression and then give up. If I reach this point, my life is on the line. Today I know I do not have to allow it to go that far.

Prayer
God, please provide me with the endurance and strength to work through my bouts with depression. Remind me that I can do something about the way that I feel. Help me remember how I have worked through my bouts in the past by hustling for the help and support that I needed. Amen

January 14

Thought for the day
It's not over till it's over.
Yogi Berra

Meditation
Many, many times I wanted it to be over. The gun, the pills, even the slower suicide of alcohol and drugs beckoned me. My depression whispered that if I would only end it all, there would be no more pain...but there also would be no more joy...no more smiles, laughter, or kisses. No more baseball games on sunny summer days, with the crack of the bats and the exciting roar of the crowd, the buttery smell of popcorn and the savory scent of hot roasted peanuts. I am grateful that I was able to remember that nothing is over until the moment I stop trying, and grateful that I was able to keep trying.

Prayer
God, grant me the strength to stay in the game and always give my best effort. Help me remember that my disease wants me dead, but you gave me life – so that I may play all my innings. Amen

January 15

Thought for the day
You may be disappointed if you fail, but you are doomed if you don't try.

Beverly Sills

Meditation
Over the years, I have experienced many disappointments in my attempt to treat my depression. I have had medicine work well for a period of time, only to have the bottom fall out later. I have been asked to switch medication on numerous occasions, and to take two different medications at the same time...medications that I was hoping to get off of soon. Each new setback has frustrated me...but what was my alternative? It was to be doomed to spiritual bankruptcy and / or death.

Prayer
God, please help me see that my disappointments are part of my recovery process. Don't let me forget that my recovery will always require effort on my part. I need to remember what the alternative will be for me if I choose to no longer get the help I need. Please continue to give me the strength to carry on. Amen

January 16

Thought for the day
The great end of life is not knowledge, but action.

Thomas Fuller

Meditation
I am unable to change my life or myself until I develop a working knowledge of both. But knowledge will avail me nothing until I act on that knowledge. This is not to say that knowledge is not important – it is. But it should be looked upon as the prerequisite to action, not as an end in and of itself. Knowledge without action will produce no effect, while action without knowledge may produce disastrous results. I feel that it is my responsibility to learn as much about my depression and the treatments that are available to me. But that alone is not enough. Using that information, I take as active a role in treating my depression as I can. I am also aware of the symptoms that indicate I am moving toward a depressive episode. With that awareness, I have a choice – I can take action and seek help, or I can do nothing. The awareness alone does not improve my situation without my taking action.

Prayer
Lord, may I be not afraid to act. May I look to you for guidance, and the strength to be an active participant in the treatment of my depression. Amen

January 17

Thought for the day
Do not dismiss your dreams. To be without dreams is to be without hope; to be without hope is to be without purpose.

Unknown

Meditation
When I am held hostage by the darkness of my depression, I am without hope and purpose. My days just stretch off endlessly into a blank gray fog, and I haven't the will or the energy to move. At these bleak times in my life, I remember my dreams, or I call a friend to help me remember. I dream of being a good parent to my children, a good spouse, and a friend among friends. I know it is possible for my dreams to come true; I have had it happen to me. The caring of my doctors and my friends have made it possible. When these things are brought into my mind with sufficient force, hope returns. I will live through this yet again. The sun will rise and the darkness will leave me. In the meantime, I can rediscover my purpose by reaching out to another who might need to remember their dreams too.

Prayer
God, make me an instrument of your will so that I may rediscover my reason for being by doing Your bidding. Let me help others, and in so doing, find my own dreams come true. Amen

January 18

Thought for the day
Blessed is he who carries within himself a god and an ideal
and who obeys it – an ideal of art, of science, or gospel
virtues. Therein lie the springs of great thoughts and great
actions.

Louis Pasteur

Meditation
One of the greatest concepts I carry within myself today is
the realization that I suffer from an *illness* called depression.
When I finally surrendered to this fact, a huge burden was
lifted off of my heart. By accepting that depression is a
treatable illness rather than believing I am a worthless,
ungrateful, hopeless waste has probably saved my life. It is
not my fault that I suffer from this illness. I did not cause it,
but…today I know that I am responsible for treating it.

Prayer
God thank you for the people you have put in my
life…people who have taught me about the disease of
depression. Help me never again believe the lies this illness
will tell. Please continue to give me the strength to fight the
good fight. Amen

January 19

Thought for the day
I don't deserve this award, but I have arthritis and I don't deserve that either.

Jack Benny

Meditation
I don't deserve to suffer from depression and neither do you. I also don't believe that God is punishing me or purposely allowing me to suffer from this illness. The greatest gifts in life have come to me as a direct result of recognizing and treating my illness, in all of its manifestations. Today I am surrounded by the love and care of many people who I would never have known had I stayed locked in the prison of depression. If I were not the person I am today, with all my struggles and imperfections, I would never need to ask anybody for help, including God...and consequently, I would end up alone once again.

Prayer
God, please help me continue to seek out your will. Thank you for opening my eyes to the rewards of living in your truths. Amen

January 20

Thought for the day
There are only two forces that unite men – fear and interest.

Napoleon Bonaparte

Meditation
Fear was my greatest motivator. It also was my greatest enemy. Before I learned about clinical depression, my fears almost led me to death. I could not stand the thought of living the rest of my life feeling the way I did. Then God put a person in my life that began to explain to me why life felt so bad. He restored some interest in life in me by convincing me that there was still hope. I united with him by making a decision to trust and follow his directions. I soon met and talked with other people that also suffered from depression. My fears have been lifted. I know that I am no longer alone.

Prayer
God thank you for putting people in my life today who know the pain that I have experienced. These people understand how it feels to have lost all hope. By bringing us together, I have overcome my fear of living and gained an interest in others. Amen

January 21

Thought for the day
When a hundred men stand together, each of them loses his mind and gets another one.

Friedrich Nietzsche

Meditation
I often talk about the influence that other recovering people have had on my life. I believe that without their help, I would not have lost my old perceptions and attitudes, and therefore would probably be institutionalized or dead today. Once I became willing to stand with others, I began to share their thoughts. In this process I have found my authentic self.

Prayer
God, please continue to give me the courage to fight the urges to isolate, and allow me to continue on my journey of recovery. Thank you for the opportunity to feel the joy and sense of belonging that has resulted from becoming united with my fellow man. Amen

January 22

Thought for the day
The chains of habit are too weak to be felt until they are too strong to be broken.

Samuel Johnson

Meditation
For years I self-medicated my depression with any and all mood altering chemicals and experiences. I would do anything to avoid feeling the pain I was in. The primary emotion I used to mask my depression was anger. In my opinion, it felt much better to be angry than to feel depressed. The problem with this approach to life is I ended up blaming the entire world for how I felt. Since I was in an active addiction with alcohol and cocaine, the spiral downward was intense. I eventually crashed and burned right into a rehabilitation center. There, I recall being told I was homicidal / suicidal. I remember thinking to myself, "How on God's green earth did I end up like this?" The shame I experienced cut straight to my heart. I soon had to accept that although my behavior was self-destructive...I knew no other way. My weak chain of habit now had become hardened steel. I no longer had the strength to break it on my own. It is only by the grace of God that I was able to receive the help I so desperately needed.

Prayer
God, help me remember who I am and where I come from. Help me remember that without my recovery, my life is nothing more than a habitual mess. Amen

January 23

Thought for the day
Oh God Thou hast created us for Thyself so that our hearts
are restless until they find their rest in thee.

St. Augustine

Meditation
Self-love is absent in the heart and mind of a person who is
in the midst of untreated, clinical depression. It is
impossible to have a loving, caring perception of oneself,
while contemplating taking your own life. Yet, without self-
love, it is impossible to care enough about ourselves to get
the help we need. Without self-love, we cannot do what we
like in life. The only event that occurred in my life that has
allowed me to begin to learn self-love, is the surrendering to
the fact that my depression is a treatable illness. Once I
accepted this fact and turned my thoughts away from the lies
this illness was telling me, I began to recover.

Prayer
God I know that you have always loved me. There have
been many days I have wondered why, yet in my heart I
know that it is true. If you, the Creator of all things, can love
me, then I must also learn to love myself. I know I cannot
love another person properly, if I first do not love myself.
Help me continue on your path of self-awareness and
discovery of self-love. Amen

January 24

Thought for the day
Be a friend to thyself, and others will be so too.

Thomas Fuller

Meditation
My life today is full because it is full of friends. My relationships I have today are the very things that continue to provide me with the strength I need to carry on. I truly believe God works through people for people. I know God talks to me through the hearts of my fellow sufferers. Some days I feel like giving up. I feel like killing my pain with any and all methods available. I know that if I did not have my circle of recovering people in my life, it would be much easier for me to concede defeat. To maintain these precious relationships, I must continue to be a friend to myself by having the willingness to forge forward into this new way of life one day at a time.

Prayer
God thank you for this new way of living. Thank you for putting me in touch with such wonderful people who are always willing to lend me their support. Amen

January 25

Thought for the day
I am not in this world to live up to your expectations.
And you are not in this world to live up to mine.
And if by chance we find each other, it's beautiful.
And if not, it can't be helped.

Unknown

Meditation
For me, nothing can send me crashing into the depths of
depression faster than guilt. If I feel I have let a friend or a
family member down, if I have failed them in some way, if I
have been less than perfect – then my disease roars into my
life with a vengeance. It magnifies my offense to titanic
proportions until I begin to believe that I am responsible for
every dreadful thing that has ever happened. But if I
remember that such bitter negativity is a result of a mental
illness and not a true picture of reality, then things begin to
change. I have to accept that I am responsible only for
treating my illness to the best of my ability each day. The
chances are very good that my subjective thought process
has made a mountain out of a molehill anyway, and the
wronged party barely remembers my "horrible" lapse. Our
friends and family love us because they choose to. We
cannot bribe or browbeat anyone into loving us. We too
have choices in whom we love. And if we find we cannot
love or be loved by a particular individual, it's not a shame
or tragedy. It is merely something we cannot control – it
can't be helped.

Prayer
God, help me remember that yours is the only perfect love.
Help me be as loving and lovable as possible – but, if I can't
please everyone, it's not a personal failure. It just can't be
helped. Amen

January 26

Thought for the day
Life is not fair. I know it isn't fair because I should be dead.

Unknown

Meditation
These two simple sentences are symbolic of my life before recovery and my life with recovery. Life was always difficult before I started to treat my depression. Today I am able to accept the fact that my life is a gift. Whenever the pressures of living begin to overwhelm me, I can always fall back on the fact that even in the midst of my most difficult times, I can still find something to be grateful for. I know that many people who suffer from clinical depression never receive any treatment. My hope is that with a stronger public awareness and sense of community among those of us who are afflicted, we may bring about the opportunity for more people to learn how to live with this illness instead of dying from it.

Prayer
God thank you for all the help I have received. Thank you for your inspiration, which has guided me in the understanding that I suffer from a potentially fatal, yet treatable illness. Amen

January 27

Thought for the day
Simplicity, simplicity, simplicity. I say, let your affairs be as two or three, and not a hundred or a thousand; instead of a million count half a dozen, and keep your accounts on your thumbnail.

Henry David Thoreau

Meditation
It is very important that I listen to what my body is telling me, especially when I am feeling the symptoms of depression. Being the compulsive-addictive type, it is very easy for me to be moving in a million different directions at one time. I can allow myself to spin my wheels so hard and fast that, before I know it, I am in too deep. My life is the most enjoyable when I am able to keep it simple, but that is not always an easy task for me. When I am slipping into a period of depression, my knee-jerk reaction is to attempt to do something outside of myself to make me feel better. What I have learned is that outside conditions really play a very small part in the make-up of my mood. It is an "inside job" so to speak. I try to keep it simple. I call a friend. I call my doctor. I pray to God.

Prayer
God, help me to keep my life simple one day at a time. Amen

January 28

Thought for the day
I deny the lawfulness of telling a lie to a sick man for fear of alarming him; you have no business with consequences, you are to tell the truth.

Samuel Johnson

Meditation
The truth is many people die from clinical depression. Many alcoholics and drug addicts are doomed to a life of active addiction because of untreated depression. The problem is that untreated depression is never listed as the cause of death in your local paper's obituary section. The paper will never write that a person died from alcoholism either. On occasion, it will state that an individual died from a drug overdose. Most of the time, all that is listed as the cause of death is "natural causes". I look with amazement, at the wonderful efforts that have been made in regard to AIDS awareness, yet I am dumbfounded by the "head in the sand" approach to depression, alcoholism, and chemical dependency. By not telling the truth concerning these illnesses, we are in fact lying to millions of sick men, women, and children.

Prayer
God, give us the strength to bring about the change that will reveal the truth. Millions of your children suffer and die, in complete isolation, because of the lack of public interest and awareness that surround these illnesses. Please help all that suffer from these maladies unite and begin to make the change. Amen

January 29

Thought for the day
Yes, 'n' how many years can some people exist
Before they're allowed to be free?
Yes. 'n' how many times can a man turn his head
Pretending he just doesn't see?
The answer, my friend is blowin' in the wind.

Bob Dylan

Meditation
I am amazed that I lived so many years in complete darkness. I can get very angry when I consider all the lost time and opportunity. There was a period in my life when I was completely ignorant of my condition. Then there was a time I was in complete denial. That was followed by a time of utter hopelessness. Finally, by the grace of God, I found the answer "blowin' in the wind', at a very special place that people who have been there, refer to as "magic mountain".

Prayer
God, please never allow me to forget where I came from. Never let me forget that I am not cured. Let me continue to learn about humility, so I may know your peace. Amen

January 30

Thought for the day
These are the times that try men's souls. The summer soldier and the sunshine patriot will, in this crisis, shrink from the service of their country, but he that stands it now, deserves the love and thanks of man and woman. Tyranny, like hell, is not easily conquered; yet we have this consolation with us, that the harder the conflict, the more glorious the triumph.

Thomas Paine

Meditation
When I read the last sentence of this quotation, I realize that I can replace the word tyranny with depression and the sentence still remains truthful and sensible. Our form of depression is not easily conquered. It is such a formidable foe because it constantly tells us we are worthless and the world would be a better place if we were no longer part of it. It is hard to muster the strength to fight when you feel like dying. Today my experiences have taught me that all I have to do is continually reach out for help. The key is to be reaching in the right direction. If I am reaching across the bar at my local tavern to treat my depression, I cannot expect much relief. In fact, in my situation, that will only intensify my depression the morning after. God, support groups, and doctors are where I can expect to begin receiving the healing I deserve. Today I can say that I do experience triumph...and it is glorious.

Prayer
God, help me remember that my recovery is a "day at a time" process. Please help me see that my depression is not easily conquered, and if I hope to have a continual reprieve from suicidal thoughts, I must treat this illness with constant vigilance. Amen

January 31

Thought for the day
Although the world is full of suffering, it is full also of overcoming it.

Helen Keller

Meditation
Let us not forget that we who suffer from depression are not alone. Let us not forget that many of our fellow sufferers have reached out and received the comfort and healing that they so desperately needed. Let us remember that our depression is an illness that must be treated. Let us separate ourselves from this illness. Let us realize that the self-defeating thoughts in our heads are the result of our untreated depression, and not a true reflection of our authentic selves.

Prayer
God, help me remember that I suffer from an illness called depression. Help me remember that you have already blessed me with doctors, medicines, and fellow sufferers who all want to help me through the dark times. Amen

February 1

Thought for the day
To be truly free, it takes more determination, courage, introspection and restraint than to be in shackles.

Pietro Bellusch

Meditation
To treat depression takes determination. It is not a once and done deal. Since I accepted my depression as an illness and began treating it, I have had numerous trips to the black hole. It can be very trying at times. I can get very discouraged at the idea that I must reach out for help yet another time. To treat depression takes courage. When I slip into the black hole, I initially experience feelings of failure. I must work through these self-defeating feelings so that I have the courage to call for help. To treat depression takes constant introspection. I have to be constantly on guard for the symptoms of this illness. The sooner I reach for help, the less painful the bout is. To treat depression takes restraint. It takes restraint not to go run and hide with a bottle of liquor, a bag of cocaine, and the shotgun. To be free from the shackles of depression requires determination, courage, introspection, and restraint.

Prayer
God, please provide me with the determination, courage, introspection, and restraint that will keep me free from the shackles of depression. Amen

February 2

Thought for the day
We who lived in concentration camps can remember the men who walked through the huts comforting others, giving away their last piece of bread. They may have been few in number, but they offer sufficient proof that everything can be taken from a man but one thing: the last of human freedoms – to choose one's attitude in any given set of circumstances – to choose one's own way.

Viktor Frankl

Meditation
How true it is. I had a friend who has since passed on, who used to say to me, "it's not what's thrown at you, it's how you catch it". I always felt like I was playing the game of life with a baseball glove that was worn and torn with the webbing missing. Every time I tried to catch one of life's line drives, it would shoot through my torn webbing and crack me right in the face. It felt that way because it was that way. I was out on the playing field alright, but I had nasty equipment. But for the grace of God, I was not allowed to quit. Somehow, I was always able to maintain hope…hope that got me to the help I needed, and showed me how to mend my glove and catch the line drives of life.

Prayer
God, please never allow me to give up hope. Help me keep your spirit of eternal life in my heart so that I may find the people who you want me to find. Help me carry the message of hope to my fellow sufferers, and encourage them to do the same. Amen

February 3

Thought for the day
Don't do things to not die, do things to enjoy living. The by-product may be not dying.

Bernie S. Siegel, M.D.

Meditation
Not dying from suicide, alcoholism, or chemical dependency was all that I hoped to achieve by getting help. Upon entering a treatment facility, I made the statement that I did not want my two sons to have to look into my coffin because I died from any or all of these maladies. I have attended enough funerals of friends who have died from these illnesses. I have seen the intense loss on their little children's faces. As I have progressed down my road of recovery, I have found that the whole experience is not about "not dying". It is about living! I am going to die...I don't know when and I don't know how. I need to leave that for my Creator to decide. My God gave me this life, and it is his decision, not mine, as to when it should end.

Prayer
God, help me seize this day. Help me live life to its fullest. Show me your wonders...teach me your ways. Help me to help others so that we may all serve you better. Amen

February 4

Thought for the day
If you won't be better tomorrow than you were today, then what do you need tomorrow for?

Rabbi Nahman of Bratslav

Meditation
Hope for a better tomorrow is a wonderful thing. The problem is that clinical depression robs us of all hope. At our worst, we curse the idea of a better tomorrow. We actually hope we never see another tomorrow again. But what about tomorrow if hope can be restored? The moment I was told that my thoughts of suicide were the result of an illness, and the illness was treatable, I began to have hope again. Today, my hopes have turned to absolute truths. I know I can get the healing I need by asking for help. I also know that although the results I hope for may not occur exactly the way I had planned, or happen within my desired time frame, the relief will come. The bout will subside.

Prayer
God, please allow me to maintain an attitude of hope. Please remind me that suicide is not natural...that it is not the answer to my perceived problems. When my life is dealing me some troublesome moments, please let me feel your presence, comfort, and peace. Amen

February 5

Thought for the day
Therefore be at peace with God, whatever you conceive him to be, and whatever your labours and aspirations, in the noisy confusion of life keep peace with your soul. With all its sham, drudgery, and broken dreams, it is still a beautiful world.

Max Ehrmann

Meditation
For us, sometimes it seemed like the only place that we'd ever find peace was in the grave. There, finally, all those hateful, hurtful voices clamoring inside our heads would be forever silenced. Of course – but we'd be dead, and one is dead for a very long time. Fortunately, we learned that there are other ways to find peace. There are concerned medical professionals. There are medications. There are kind friends who understand what we are feeling and who can show us how to deal with our feelings. There are Twelve Step programs for those of us who need them. All we have to do is make the smallest effort and help is on the way. We can regret the past – all the shame and drudgery, the wasted opportunities, days spent mired in the muck of our disease – or we can enjoy the peace of today – a quiet moment, a rosy dawn, a fiery red sunset, a child's laugh. There is much beauty out there for us, if we take care of ourselves first. Treat the illness of depression, and you will find the peace and contentment you are meant to have.

Prayer
God grant us peace. Amen

February 6

Thought for the day
Give me neither poverty nor riches; feed me with food convenient for me.

Proverbs 30:8

Meditation
I have spent enormous amounts of time and energy trying to create an external environment that would make me feel good. I really believed that if only I had...love, money, power...you can fill in the blanks, I would feel successful and whole. All my efforts to achieve financial independence for example were for naught. The size of my bank account never really had anything to do with how I felt about myself. What I really needed was some new information, some guidance and inspiration. The Bible often refers to the word of God as food for the soul. The point is that I had a hole in my soul that was never going to get filled unless I started filling it with the right things. Thank God I found the help I needed.

Prayer
God, guide me toward your wisdom and inspiration. Help me remember that I cannot maintain a spiritual condition that is conducive to recovery without you and other recovering people in my life. Amen

February 7

Thought for the day
Life is better than death, I believe, if only because it is less boring and because it has fresh peaches in it.

Thomas Walker

Meditation
I have spent a lot of time contemplating death. I have also considered and attempted taking my own life. I can tell you that when you're drunk, sitting in your car with the exhaust pumping into your vehicle, it just doesn't feel like God's will. I have escaped death on numerous occasions. Today, I have accepted that I need to leave my final moment in this realm in the hands of my Creator. Nature does abhor a suicide. I believe life is supposed to be as simple and as enjoyable as fresh peaches...but if I'm not treating my depression, all I'll ever have is the "pits".

Prayer
God, help me be grateful when I can no longer think of one reason to live another moment. Help me see that in the scope of things, my problems are not the end of the world. Help me remember that suicide is absolutely the most selfish action that any person can take. Help me find the "fresh peaches" that you have provided for me. Help me to relax. Amen

February 8

Thought for the day
Life is a long lesson in humility.
Sir James M. Barrie

Meditation
For me, humility is nothing more than being honest with myself and knowing where I end and God begins. Life is so wonderful when I am able to see God's presence in my life. The problem I have is that I so often stop looking toward God, and then to my amazement, he is nowhere to be found. It usually goes something like this. "God thank you for your help getting me here. Now I'll take over. I'll see you later". And off I go to conquer the world. The end result is usually a feeling of emptiness. Once I return to the "walk", which I believe is God's will for me, I begin to feel worthwhile, whole, and complete.

Prayer
God, help me remember that in the past, when I have allowed my ego to edge you out, I have ended up lost. Please shepherd me and keep me in your flock. Provide me with the compassion to always be a channel of your peace. Amen

February 9

Thought for the day
Nurture strength of spirit to shield you in sudden misfortune. But do not distress yourself with imaginings. Many fears are born of fatigue and loneliness. Beyond a wholesome discipline, be gentle with yourself.

Max Ehrmann

Meditation
As a person with a chronic illness, I need to listen especially closely to my body. I must be aware of being tired and hungry. When my muscles ache and my stomach growls, my mind follows and begins to dwell on the things that are wrong with my life instead of what's right. Before I learned about this body/mind link, I would push myself physically past the point of fatigue and then wonder why I felt so rotten! If I kept pushing, I found myself back in the pit of fear and despair. We must learn to be kind to ourselves, to put us first as often as possible. We have to eat and sleep well. We have to nurture ourselves, to build the health we need to sustain those we love and ourselves. When we are depressed, the last thing we want to do is care for our body and spirit. That is the time when we call our doctors and our friends. They will take care of us until we can care for ourselves.

Prayer
God, help me love myself the way I know you love me. Help me remember that you don't create junk. I am worthy of myself, and I must treat myself with care. Amen

February 10

Thought for the day
The real reason for not committing suicide is because you always know how swell life gets again after the hell is over.

Ernest Hemingway

Meditation
How sweet life is after the hell is over. How difficult it is to see the light when you're in hell, though. It is the work that I do outside the black hole that prepares me for when I slip in it again. I have pulled myself out enough times now to know that life will get "swell" again. Get the help you need. Do not be afraid. Build a support group that you can truly count on. Build a group that truly understands. Realize that you suffer from a disease called depression. You can stop beating yourself up now. You can begin to be gentle with yourself. Everything will be fine. Just don't try to get better on your own. Depression is an illness that wants to isolate you and then kill you. Please, when you are suffering, do not allow yourself to be alone.

Prayer
God, please give all of us who suffer from clinical depression the wisdom to understand that we have an illness and that there is help available. Help us all have the courage and strength to ask for help. Strip us of our shame. Rid us of our false pride. Help us fight the good fight. Amen

February 11

Thought for the day
There are days when it takes all you've got just to keep up with the losers.

Robert Orpen

Meditation
It is very important to keep our expectations of ourselves in tune with reality. I will so often set myself up for failure by expecting too much from myself...especially when I am having a bout with depression. I have to accept this illness with all the limitations that it can, from time to time, put on me. I really do not believe that any person is a loser like this quote says. But the spirit of the thought is that some days we can only do the best we can with what we have. Life deals the cards; we have to play them. The great thing is if our hand is all sevens and below without any pairs, we can fold and play another hand. Even the worst of players will eventually draw a pair of aces.

Prayer
God, please continue to see me through the storms of life. Help me see that there is always someone who has it worse than I do. Give me the wisdom to see that there is truly always something to be grateful for. Help me find the strength to keep up with whatever life has to offer, especially in the down times. Amen

February 12

Thought for the day
Life consists in what a man is thinking of all day.
Ralph Waldo Emerson

Meditation
When I spend my day worrying about what time the bullet store closes or if the plug to the toaster will reach the tub, it is safe to say that my life is consisting of suicidal thoughts. Of course at this point, there should be all types of bells and whistles going off in my head, alerting me that I should be calling for help. Beyond that, this is a hell of a way to live life. As it is written in the good book, my mind is like a garden. I must constantly weed it of thoughts that are counterproductive to a fruitful and plentiful harvest. If I want to enjoy the fruits of life, I must have a mind that is well cultivated. I may have to ask for help to achieve the results I desire. I will definitely have to consider whether any of my old thoughts have provided me with a worthwhile yield in the past.

Prayer
God, please provide me with the intestinal fortitude and tenacity to rid my mind of counterproductive thoughts. I know I cannot be available to do your will if my mind is filled with weeds. Amen

February 13

Thought for the day
Growth is the only evidence of life.
Cardinal Newman

Meditation
Spiritual growth is of the utmost importance if we hope to sustain a successful life. Today, I am acutely aware of the fact that some of my greatest setbacks have given way to my largest spurts of growth. To stand still and not attempt to recover from our setbacks is spiritual bankruptcy. The dilemma is that clinical depression robs us of so many things. One of those things is our spirituality. But I say to you, do not be discouraged. If you recognize your bankruptcy as another symptom of this illness, you will be better armed to fight. And to have some fight left is growth!

Prayer
God, please provide me with the spiritual nourishment I need to continue growing. Help me remember that my growth does not have to occur overnight. Help me be patient with myself while I am living through the process. Amen

February 14

Thought for the day
The tragedy of life is not so much what men suffer, but rather what they miss.

Thomas Carlyle

Meditation
How many precious moments in my life have I missed due to my depression? How many years of my life did I waste on a barstool trying to kill the pain of my otherwise miserable existence? I can remember my children trying to wake me up in the early afternoon after I was coming off a two-day alcohol / cocaine run. They wanted me to play ball with them. I remember my heart wishing that I could get up off the couch and go play with them, but I couldn't because I was so depressed. The shame that I felt was overwhelming. I remember thinking that I was such a terrible dad. I really started to believe that my wife and children would be much happier and much better off, if I were no longer in the picture. I was in such great pain. Thank God, I finally got help. I can truthfully say that when I reflect on the things I lost prior to receiving treatment for my depression, alcoholism, and cocaine addiction…I grieve.

Prayer
God thank you so much for the many blessings I have experienced since I began on this road of recovery. I am so grateful I have been given the opportunity to share my story with others, in the hope that they may also find comfort in your saving grace. Amen

February 15

Thought for the day
The man who has no inner life is the slave of his surroundings.

Henri Frederic Amiel

Meditation
When I was at my lowest point, I was a shell of a man. There was nothing left inside of me except pain, hate, and discontent. I literally had to fight like hell to sit upright in a chair. All I wanted to do was crumble into a dark corner and die. When I was younger, life was easier to bounce back from. As my illness was left untreated, life seemed to push me down deeper and deeper into the black hole. I found it more and more difficult to recover from life's low points. I slowly lost all faith in myself and in God. Worse yet, I became very certain that God had lost all faith in me. Because I had no inner-self, no authentic center of reference regarding who I was, I had no choice but to rely on my surroundings to define me. When a man is forced into this level of existence, he is doomed to a shallow, spiritually bankrupt, meaningless life.

Prayer
God, please give me the strength to continue my journey within. Grant me the honesty that I need for accurate self-appraisal. Surround me with people who can give me the constructive criticism I will need to stay on my path of recovery. Grant me the willingness to remain open-minded long enough to hear what they have to say. Amen

February 16

Thought for the day
Everyday...begin the first thing in the morning to consider how you can bring a real joy to someone else.

Dr. Alfred Adler

Meditation
At first this may seem like an insult. "Hey, I'm the sick person", we exclaim. Why should we want to bring happiness to others when we seem to have so little of it ourselves? The nature of our illness is to isolate us. We turn away from those who love us. We feel unworthy of their concern and affection. We feel less than human. By actively taking steps to think of others, to think of how we can bring them pleasure, we are pulled up and out of our diseased thinking and into the light and warmth of right relationships. And it isn't long before we find that the happiness we can bring to others is exceeded only by the happiness we feel in delighting our friends and family. Smiles and laughter are very contagious.

Prayer
God, I know you did not put me on this earth to be miserable. You did not bring me along this far to be a failure. Help me live today according to your will, and to brighten the lives of those who love me. Amen

February 17

Thought for the day
Go placidly amid the noise and the haste, and remember what peace there may be in silence. As far as possible without surrender, be on good terms with all persons. Speak your truth quietly and clearly, and listen to others, even the dull and ignorant; they too have their story. Be yourself. Especially do not feign affection. Neither be cynical about love – for in the face of all aridity and disenchantment it is as perennial as the grass. Take kindly the counsel of the years, gracefully surrendering the things of youth. Nurture strength of spirit to shield you in sudden misfortune. But do not distress yourself with imaginings. Many fears are born of fatigue and loneliness. Beyond a wholesome discipline, be gentle with yourself. You are a child of the universe no less than the trees and the stars; you have a right to be here. And whether or not it is clear to you, no doubt the universe is unfolding as it should. Therefore be at peace with God, whatever you conceive Him to be, and whatever your labours and aspirations, in the noisy confusion of life keep peace with your soul. With all its sham, drudgery and broken dreams, it is still a beautiful world

Desiderata

Meditation
Peace be still.

Prayer
God, grant me the serenity, to accept the things I cannot change. The courage to change the things I can, and the wisdom to know the difference. Amen

February 18

Thought for the day
Loneliness and the feeling of being unwanted is the most terrible poverty.

Mother Teresa

Meditation
Loneliness and the feeling of being unwanted are two feelings that we who suffer from this illness are all too familiar with. We must remember that both are definitely symptoms of clinical depression and should not be taken lightly. When I am having a bout with depression, It is not uncommon for me to feel completely isolated and alone even in the midst of many people. I can often become resentful and jealous of other people's seemingly happy lives. I wonder why I can't be more like them. These feelings lead to the feeling of being unwanted, less than, and worthless. This in turn leads to "better off dead". As Mother Teresa's quote says, this "is the most terrible poverty". It is of the utmost importance that we learn to recognize these feelings as symptoms of an illness and not as our authentic selves. Then we must get help.

Prayer
God, please grant me the inspiration to realize that I am not junk. Please help me find your spirit within me so that I have the strength to fight back the wave of lies that my illness will tell me. Help me remember that my illness is real and it wants to isolate and kill me. Please light my path and guide me toward serenity and peace. Amen

February 19

Thought for the day
Love is the irresistible desire to be desired irresistibly.
Louis Ginsberg

Meditation
How desperate have we been in our attempts to feel loved? How difficult has it been for our companions to convince us that we are special, beautiful people who have so much to contribute to life? How can we possibly love when we are filled with so much self-contempt? Usually, the first person that I will try to blame for how I feel is my wife. What I have learned in my recovery process is that nobody can make anybody feel any certain way. I have also learned that when I am in the midst of depression, I am going to feel depressed. By accepting that my depression is the result of a treatable illness and not some character flaw on my part, or the result of somebody else's actions or lack of action, I can let myself, my wife, and anybody else that I might be blaming, off the hook. It's just not their fault. I like to feel irresistibly desired, but I must remember that I can't feel that way with a shotgun in my mouth. It is absolutely impossible to feel loved and be contemplating taking your own life at the same time. By treating my illness, one day at a time, I am now able to feel loved.

Prayer
God, help me continue to grow toward self-love so I may be able to love others – and accept their love in return. Your words say that I am to love others as I love myself, but when I feel like taking my own life...what then? Help me remember that my spiritual growth occurs from within my soul and my ability to love and to be loved will always be in direct proportion to my ability to love myself. Amen

February 20

Thought for the day
Doctors are busy playing God when so few of us have the qualifications. And besides, the job is taken.

Bernie S. Siegel, MD

Meditation
Today I have a strong faith in the healing powers of my God. I believe God has seen me through some of my darkest hours. I have faith that God never abandoned me even though I had given up on Him. I do not need to know why I am afflicted with my current maladies. Whenever I become frustrated about my condition all I need to do is look at the world that surrounds me. There are so many who have it so much worse. When my depression tells me that my life is worthless and I should die, I can counter that lie with a quick glance at the human atrocities that are occurring at any given moment in our country and throughout the world. I also believe that my God works through people for people. I believe God has blessed me with modern medicine and skilled physicians. I am blind if I do not accept all the help that God has placed before me.

Prayer
God thank you for the many blessings you have bestowed upon me. Thank you for the doctors and medicines that are so readily available to me. Please help all of mankind work towards providing the medical care that so many of the world's population is in need of. You have provided enough food, clothing, and medicines for all of your children, yet, because of our selfishness, many needy people live without what we take for granted. Help us all learn to share a little better. Amen

February 21

Thought for the day
Man should not strive to eliminate his complexes, but to get in accord with them; they are legitimately what directs his contact in the world.

Sigmund Freud

Meditation
At some point in my recovery process, I completely surrendered to the fact that I suffered from alcoholism, chemical dependency, and clinical depression. I also accepted the fact that I would never be able to completely rid myself of these maladies. I finally realized I had but two alternatives; die from these illnesses, or die with these illnesses. Today I prefer the latter. I have become in accord with my complexes in the sense that I acknowledge the authenticity of them all. By doing so, I have been able to begin a recovery process that legitimately directs my contact with this world. My life is so rewarding today because I am able to share my experience, strength, and hope with so many people. More importantly, I am now able to learn from other people's experiences and apply their shared wisdom to my own life.

Prayer
God, please help me be honest with myself. Sometimes I do get discouraged and feel like giving into these illnesses. Sometimes I feel like I am just spinning my wheels and not really getting anywhere. Help me accept the fact that every day I maintain continuous sobriety and do not attempt suicide, I have grown. Please help me continue to learn how to live with these illnesses so that I do not have to die from them. Amen

February 22

Thought for the day
I was sick, and ye visited me.

Matthew 25:36

Meditation
It is only by the grace of God that I am alive and sober today. For years I tried to stay sober but continued to show up drunk. Then, after I had given up all hope of ever achieving continuous sobriety, I was diagnosed with clinical depression. I remember thinking that I could not handle yet another problem. My alcoholism and cocaine addiction was severe enough, now to add depression onto my plate was unthinkable in my estimation. Yet today I believe that diagnosis to have been my saving grace. I believe my sobriety is contingent on the daily maintenance of my spiritual condition. The level of spirituality I need to maintain on a daily basis cannot be achieved when I am in the midst of depression. It is absolutely impossible. So it is a matter of life and death that I treat my depression one day at a time. I also must remember that I cannot treat my depression if I am drinking and using cocaine. That combination will eventually lead to more depression and thus throw the entire vicious cycle back into play. I believe when we are ready to give up fighting and accept God's answers to our problems, our prayers are both heard and answered.

Prayer
God, during my darkest hours you cared for me because I could not care for myself. Now that I have been returned to reasonable health, I so often revert back to my old way of thinking. Please help me maintain the balance in my life that will allow me to continue my spiritual growth. Amen

February 23

Thought for the day
Ask many of us who are disabled what we would like in life
and you would be surprised how few would say, 'Not to be
disabled.' We accept our limitations.

Itzhak Perlman

Meditation
My recovery has taught me that I do have limitations today.
This has been very hard for me to accept, and honestly, I still
occasionally struggle with it. You see I am a perfectionist
who is brutally hard on himself. When I am in the middle of
a bout with depression, I can become very impatient and
dissatisfied with myself. I feel like I should not feel the way
I do. What a recipe for disaster this self-defeating thinking
can be. It is a humbling process for me to accept that my
maladies can be disabling from time to time. Sometimes all
I can hope for is to just get by for another moment. But the
question remains, would I choose not to be a depression
suffering, alcoholic, and cocaine addict today? The truth is
that sometimes I wish I did not have to deal with it. There
are other times though, that I am so grateful for the many
good things that my condition has brought into my life.

Prayer
God thank you for seeing me through my darkest hours and
delivering me into this new way of life. Help me not to get
discouraged or feel sorry for myself. Help me keep the faith.
Amen

February 24

Thought for the day
If a man does not keep pace with his companions, perhaps it is because he hears a different drummer. Let him step to the music which he hears, however measured or far away.
Henry David Thoreau

Meditation
I am better off when I am not comparing myself to the world that surrounds me. The reason I do not have the luxury of this point of reference is because my perceptions of reality can be very distorted from time to time. I am also reminded that people's outsides frequently do not match their insides, so the comparisons are dishonest to begin with. When I am scrambling to determine whether I measure up, I am setting myself up for a major let down. I am no longer being grateful for what I have because I am so busy noting all I am lacking. It is difficult for me to feel happy, joyous, and free when I feel like I have been deprived of all the joys others seemingly possess. Upon closer examination, It is usually revealed to me that, although I do not "have it all", I certainly do have enough. The greatest joy I have is when I am happy with who I am.

Prayer
God, help me be myself. Remind me that I do not have rise to anyone's expectations but my own, and my expectations need to be based within the realm of reality. Amen

February 25

Thought for the day
They are able who think they are able.
Virgil

Meditation
Why not you? Millions of men and women are recovering from clinical depression. They come from all walks of life. Rich, poor, black and white, and every color in between. Christian, Jew, Atheist, man, woman, child. They all have fought the fight. They have all won the race. They refused to accept that their life could never get better. Somewhere deep within themselves, they found that ray of hope that beckoned them to call for help. You do deserve to get well too.

Prayer
God, please guide all the lost children in the direction of hope. Help them not give up on life. Show them the way to recovery so they may then help others. Amen

February 26

Thought for the day
It's the whole, not the detail, that matters.

German proverb

Meditation
I have expended a great deal of energy over the course of my life trying to figure out why I am the way I am. I have anguished over the details and events of my past, trying desperately to make sense out of them all. I was once under the illusion that by having my life all figured out...it would somehow become easier to live. After years of research and therapy I have finally concluded that knowing where I came from is necessary in helping me define in what direction I should now go...but this knowledge will not propel me there on its own. What I have learned is that understanding the events and circumstances that have shaped me, will not automatically change me. How I feel about something is actually of greater importance than the event itself. And the greatest freedom of all is to now be able to exercise my right to choose how I feel about anything...past, present, and future. It is the action that follows the awareness that really matters.

Prayer
God, help me keep my eyes clearly focused on your goals. Please help me let go of my desire to analyze and dissect, and show me how to just be. Amen

February 27

Thought for the day
Longevity is having a chronic disease and taking care of it.
Oliver Wendell Holmes, Jr.

Meditation
Untreated clinical depression kills people. It is a chronic yet treatable disease that destroys the lives of those who suffer and devastates all that come into contact with its prey. When a loved one commits suicide, all who are left behind have to deal with the confusion and pain. They try to make sense out of it all. They think that maybe they had something to do with it. Children suffer the most. If Daddy or Mommy kills himself or herself, the child will inevitably have some feelings of responsibility to varying degrees. For all of us who suffer from this illness, there lies an awesome responsibility to take care of ourselves one day at a time. To enjoy a great span of life is the goal...not to leave a legacy of pain and grief for those who love us.

Prayer
God, help me help myself for others, until I am able to help myself for self. Squelch the self-defeating thoughts that tell me I have no value to anyone, and lift me to my feet so I may go find the help I need to take care of this chronic disease. Amen

February 28

Thought for the day
Have patience with all things, but chiefly have patience with
yourself. Do not lose courage in considering your own
imperfections, but instantly set about remedying them –
every day begin the task anew.

St. Francis de Sales

Meditation
Patience and courage are two essential attributes that
depression will steal away from us. We must accept and
understand that depression will, by its very nature, take away
our will to live. How then are we to be patient and
courageous in the midst of the black hole? My experience
has taught me that adopting a new attitude toward my illness
has been key to my continual survival. Today I know what
depression feels like. I also know that it is capable of taking
my life. I must consistently separate myself from this illness
and instantly set about remedying the symptoms. By
surviving the black hole, by finding renewal and hope
through working with my friends in recovery and members
of the medical community, I can now begin every day the
task anew.

Prayer
God thank you for the continual renewal of patience,
courage, and hope. Please help me always remember that
my depression is an illness, and the messages that it tells me
are nothing more than the symptoms of that illness, and not
my authentic self. Amen

March 1

Thought for the day
Responsibility n: A detachable burden easily shifted to the shoulders of God, Fate, Fortune, Luck or one's neighbor. In the days of astrology it was customary to unload it upon a star.

Ambrose Bierce

Meditation
How often have we laid helpless waiting for somebody or something to come strolling along and make it all better for us? How often have we prayed to God to help us while we were not doing anything to help ourselves? I believe my prayers will never be answered if my actions do not correspond with my requests. I believe God can move mountains, but I must bring the shovel. I do not believe my depression is a detachable burden that I can pass off as someone else's responsibility. It is my life, my recovery, and I am 100% responsible for the actions I choose to take today. God, Fate, Fortune, Neighbors, and even Luck may and will play a role in my success, but if I am not actively pursuing their assistance, my success will be limited if not non-existent.

Prayer
God thank you for the awareness of the responsibility I have to take care of myself. Thank you for teaching me that anything in my life that is of any true value does require a level of effort on my part. Amen

March 2

Thought for the day
During acute depression, avoid trying to set your whole life in order at once. If you take on assignments so heavy that you are sure to fail in them at the moment, then you are allowing yourself to be tricked by your unconscious. Thus you will continue to make sure of your failure, and when it comes, you will have another alibi for still more retreat into depression. In short, the 'all or nothing' attitude is a most destructive one. It is best to begin with whatever the irreducible minimums of activity are. Then work for an enlargement of these – day by day.

Bill W., cofounder of AA

Meditation
There are days when, in spite of all my efforts, getting out of bed is my biggest accomplishment. It is on such days when my depression can easily worsen as I look around at all the undone tasks – the unwashed dishes, the unmade beds, the unreturned phone calls, the overdue report. It would be so easy to hate myself for the mess I've made. But I have to remind myself that everyday I battle a disease, and like any chronic sufferer, I will have good days and bad days. Today I got out of bed. Perhaps tomorrow I will make the bed. We can strive only for progress, not perfection. If we need help, we only need to ask. The messes will wait until we can attend to them. They always do.

Prayer
God, help me remember to be kind to myself first, one day at a time. Amen

March 3

Thought for the day
I'm alone,
Yeah, I don't know if I can face the night.

Aerosmith

Meditation
Though I might feel depressed at this time, it is only one moment in eternity. I have accumulated tools in my toolbox from life experiences that I can now use. I can look at my past depression, inventory it, and use the tool or tools that I have used in the past to pull myself out of the darkness of despair. The weight of a lifetime is too much to carry, but I can break it down into one day, or even one hour or one second if need be. I must tell myself that this will not last forever.

Prayer
God, please give me the strength to cope with my current depression. Please help me to keep this one moment in perspective within the entire scheme of my life. Amen

March 4

Thought for the day
Never think that God's delays are God's denials. Hold on; hold fast; hold out. Patience is genius.

Comte de Buffon

Meditation
How often have we prayed for God to do our will, with little or no concern as to whether our desires complied with his will? How often do we pray for something and then go out and "make it happen"? We just force our will onto somebody or something and reconcile that it must be God's will because, after all, our intentions were good and we do know what is best for other people as well as for ourselves. And then things don't turn out as expected. Something occurs that was a nasty surprise and we find ourselves angry with God. Why did he let this happen? If only God would have followed my plan, all would be well. The truth is that I have no idea what God has in store for me today. And if I don't know what God has in store for me, how can I possibly know what he has in store for you? I must have faith. That is all there is to it. God's plan for me may be entirely different than my own. I always learn this soon enough because any time I am operating outside of God's will, I pay a spiritual price. God does answer my prayers, but not always on my time schedule, and sometimes he says NO! Some of my greatest spiritual experiences have been the result of a NO! God Speed.

Prayer
God, please help me remember that you are always present and working in my life. Please help me accept and understand that sometimes your plans for me are to serve, not to be served. Amen

March 5

Thought for the day
The fewer the words, the better the prayer.
Martin Luther

Meditation
God please help me find the help I so desperately need.

Prayer
God thank you. Amen

March 6

Thought for the day
Religion without science is lame; science without religion is blind.

Albert Einstein

Meditation
Science is constantly discovering new, innovative forms of treatment for a host of illnesses. It is only in the second half of this century that science has begun to unveil suitable medical treatments for depression. How fortunate we are to live in this era of modern medicine, and how foolish we would be not to take advantage of it. I truly believe that God works through people, for people. We are all in this thing together. God has blessed some men and women with the intellect and intestinal fortitude to find the causes and cures for so many illnesses. As a result, we who suffer from depression can find relief from this otherwise hideous, potentially fatal malady. If you are suffering, call your doctor or a close friend who understands. If you're not suffering at the present time, be the friend that somebody else can call.

Prayer
God thank you for the people you have put in my life that have helped me save it. I was feeling utterly hopeless, convinced that the only thing left for me to do was die. Then a man told me about depression. He told me this illness wants me to isolate and die. He told me to get up off the couch and be with people who care. He told me to see a doctor. Thank you! Amen

March 7

Thought for the day
We will either find a way, or make one.

Hannibal

Meditation
We need to have a fierce determination not to succumb to our depression and die. What a difficult task it is to fight when you have no fight left. But by practicing new behaviors and belief systems, we have the reinforcement that we may well need to see us through our next bout with depression. I feel as though I am constantly preparing myself for my next inevitable low. I no longer expect not to experience the symptoms of my maladies. I consider them part of my life. That does not mean for one minute that I should or will surrender to them. It is by knowing them that I am able to fight for what I do deserve...recovery. I can say that I have made many mistakes trying to find my way. I can also say, with certainty, that there are many more mistakes to follow. But the action and desire to change my life has had such a positive impact on me, that the action alone is all I need to keep me alive another day.

Prayer
God, please continue to provide me with the courage and hope to change today. Help me be gentle with myself. I know I will make mistakes along the way, so please continue to guide me along your chosen path. Amen

March 8

Thought for the day
Get your facts first, and then you can distort 'em as much as you please.

Mark Twain

Meditation
For years I survived with depression in complete ignorance. I had no information whatsoever concerning this illness. I felt so different, so messed up in the head, bordering on insanity. Then, by the grace of God, I started to learn the facts. I began to look back on my life, and I could see that I had been suffering from clinical depression since my early teens. Today, with the help of my support group, I feel as though I have enough facts to adequately recognize my symptoms, and then get the help that I need. Yet, every once in awhile, I want to deny the authenticity of this illness and begin finding a person, place, or thing to blame for my feeling depressed. If I am contemplating suicide it is because some person, place, or thing has hurt me so badly that I must kill myself, right? Does that not sound completely insane? It should because it is. Distorting the facts about depression is yet another symptom that we who suffer must be aware of. Our lives may depend on it.

Prayer
God, please help me remain honest with myself. Denial will eventually kill me. Whether it is in regard to my alcoholism, chemical dependency, or depression, I must remain honest about the authenticity of these illnesses. Amen

March 9

Thought for the day
Depression is the inability to construct a future.
Rollo May

Meditation
For all of us who have experienced the darkness of the black hole, how could depression be anything other than the inability to construct a future? When depressed, it is impossible for me to have any worthwhile, positive, hopeful thoughts for the future. It is actually the future that I dread the most because, from the vantage point of the black hole, there is no future worth living for. This is why it is so important to reach out for help when I am depressed. Left to my own devices, I might self-destruct. But with the help of an understanding friend or physician, I am able to see my way out of the darkness and into the light of the future.

Prayer
God, please help me to keep my eye on your shining light. Help me to understand that there is no future for me if I don't take care of myself by treating my depression. My hopes and dreams can only materialize outside of the darkness, so please continue to guide me toward your light. Amen

March 10

Thought for the day
Life is like a game of cards. The hand that is dealt you represents determinism; the way you play it is free will.

Jawaharlal Nehru

Meditation
I believe that I was dealt alcoholism, chemical dependency, and depression. I know that there has been, and will continue to be, countless hours of debate as to whether there is a biological predisposition that sets up these illnesses, or if they are acquired by a wide range of abuse and misfortune. The truth is perhaps somewhere in the middle. My point is what difference does it make? They are the cards that I am now holding. Whether I was dealt them, or got them on a draw, they are now my responsibility to play. Perhaps I am victim to a poor shuffler and dealer? In my opinion, Mom the "shuffler" and Dad the "dealer" probably should not have been allowed to play cards, but that's another story. Today I have accepted that there should be no more whining and complaining...no more finger pointing and name-calling. It's my life now. It is yours, too!

Prayer
God, help me get over feeling like a victim...help me take personal responsibility for my recovery and my life. Amen

March 11

Thought for the day
The trouble with the rat race is that even if you win, you're
still a rat.

Lily Tomlin

Meditation
Sometimes I just need to slow down. To put that concept in
more personal, laser specific terminology, I need to stop my
battleship mind from getting ahead of my rowboat ass. I
believe we are all guilty of occasionally taking ourselves a
little too seriously. If you think about it, when we are in the
black hole, we are taking ourselves extremely seriously.
And so we should because, if we have limited knowledge of
our condition, or have not even begun to accept depression
as an illness, our lives are on the line. But, if we have been
receiving treatment and have a strong support system, if we
have been through enough bouts to know that we will get
through the next one, then we can excuse ourselves from our
self-designed rat race and just relax. "This too shall pass"
can be our motto as we take care of ourselves through the
dark moments of our lives.

Prayer
God, please let me find the peace that will exceed all
understanding. Please nurture and protect me when I am
experiencing dark times in my life. Amen

March 12

Thought for the day
I have fought a good fight, I have finished my course, I have kept the faith.

2 Timothy 4:7

Meditation
When you feel like you have had enough of life...carry on. When you feel like your life is a complete waste...carry on. When you feel like there is not one person who understands your pain...carry on. When you feel like you have no more fight left, that you are about to go under for the final time...carry on. Keep the faith, my friend. Remember that you are no longer alone. There are millions of us all around you. We all want to help you. We do not want you to die from this illness. Finish the course. Call for help. Scream for help. Search forever for the peace that is awaiting you. We will love you until you can love yourself. And once you can love yourself...go love somebody else.

Prayer
God, help me feel the love and support that surrounds me. Help me remember that you are always present in my life, especially during my darkest moments. Amen

March 13

Thought for the day
The whole head is sick, and the whole heart faint.
Isaiah 1:5

Meditation
Does this accurately describe our state of being when we are fighting depression? God knows that my whole head was sick. When I look back at the thought processes that I had when I was depressed, the screams for self-destruction, the feelings of utter worthlessness...I realize how desperately sick I was. When I am having an episode with depression, I cannot trust my own thinking or my perception of myself. I must also remember that my depression will wither away my heart. It is very difficult to maintain a strong heart, and a strong faith in God and my fellow man, when I'm at my low points. When my heart becomes faint, I am dangerously close to taking my life. But the good news is that I no longer have to live like that. I recognize the symptoms of my illness, accept them as real, and get the healing that I need. If you are currently struggling to sort through your depression, get more help please. You are important, and we do need you.

Prayer
God, please strengthen all the hearts of my fellow sufferers, so that they too, may maintain the strength of heart that is necessary to see them through the times of the "sick head".
Amen

March 14

Thought for the day
Be not deceived; God is not mocked: for whatsoever a man soweth, that shall he also reap.

Galatians 6:7

Meditation
It is when our depression is in remission that we must sow. God did not save us from drowning just to watch us smash against the rocks of the shore, but that is exactly what will happen to us if we become complacent and just lazily float upon tranquil times. By helping others, I feel that I am part of life. I feel that I am making a difference. We must always be looking for soil in which we may sow the seeds of God's everlasting love. By helping our fellow sufferers, we sow, and then reap the rewards of living a purposeful life.

Prayer
God, please continue to show me where I end and you begin. Thank you for guiding me in a direction that allows me to live yet another day to sow your seeds of love. Amen

March 15

Thought for the day
Two roads diverged in a wood and I –
I took the one less traveled by,
And that has made all the difference.

Robert Frost

Meditation
I was lost in the darkness of the darkest forest. I do not understand exactly why I chose the road less traveled and got help for myself. What I do believe is that I am truly blessed to still be alive. Most people who suffer from depression never get the help they deserve. Some will begin, and then quit. It is not because they are quitters. It is because they are exhibiting yet another symptom of the illness. Depression tells us we might as well give up because we are no good or undeserving of any other life than the dark, miserable existence that we have become accustomed to. Despite how I got here, here I am. And here you are: reading these words, contemplating how you arrived at this point and considering the options that you have for the rest of your life. The choice of making the effort will continue to make all the difference in our lives and all the lives that we set out to touch.

Prayer
God thank you for your continuous, unconditional love. I know I will never understand all the happenings in this world that are a result of your will. I will never fully understand why I have been allowed to live such a rich life while some of my brothers and sisters have already been called home to you. Please help me to honor your many gifts by living a life that is pleasing to you. Amen

March 16

Thought for the day
Don't compromise yourself. You are all you've got.

Janis Joplin

Meditation
Your life is a precious, fragile moment that is completely unrepeatable by any other spirit to come. Within you there lives a spirit that must be heard. It will continue to love beneath all your rage, beneath all your tears, beneath all your fears, it will never die. Help yourself to live by the whispers of your spirit. Help us to hear your spirit's softness. Share with us your spirit's joy. All that we search for in life, our spirit holds buried underneath the wreckage of our failed explorations. Never compromise yourself.

Prayer
God, please teach me how to love and nurture myself. You know that I have spent much of my life searching in vain for that "magic something" that would make me feel "good". I have always returned from my journey sorely disappointed and a bit more hardened toward this world in which I live. Help me understand that my search is over once I allow your spirit to embrace mine. Amen

March 17

Thought for the day
I believe that this neglected, wounded, inner child of the past
is the major source of human misery.

John Bradshaw

Meditation
Many of us who suffer from depression are dually
diagnosed, meaning that we also suffer from alcoholism and
/ or chemical dependency. Some of us also are a byproduct
of an abusive childhood. I happen to be all of the above.
What this means to me is that I need to be working on my
recovery in a variety of ways. I cannot treat my depression if
I am pouring a depressant down my throat all night long at
the corner pub. Neither is it effective for me to attempt to
stay sober if I am miserable and heartsick. I am not very
concerned with the cause of my situations. I have a pretty
good idea how I ended up the way I did, but knowledge of
what happened has never once eased the pain or changed the
past. The question that we all need to ask ourselves is "what
are we going to do about it"? To recover from a neglected,
wounded childhood requires the person in the mirror to make
a decision to no longer accept the lies of their youth, and get
help. To learn how to live a happy, productive lifestyle with
the illness of depression requires the same person to reach
out again and again until they find the relief that they are
looking for.

Prayer
God, for many of us, our problems seem so insurmountable
that we never really make a strong effort at changing our
lives because we just do not know where to begin. Help us
to relax and take that first step toward recovery by asking
somebody for help. Remind us that our recovery will be a
process, not an event. Amen

March 18

Thought for the day
Never let your head hang down. Never give up and sit down and grieve. Find another way. And don't pray when it rains if you don't pray when the sun shines.

Satchel Paige

Meditation
My life has been filled with "foxhole" prayers. When I have been down and out or in any type of trouble, I have turned to God and asked for forgiveness and pardon. Eventually, the problem would pass and I would soon forget the promises that I made during my time of need. It is very important for me to remember to give thanks to God on the sunny days. By doing so, I strengthen my spiritual condition, which in turn, allows me to refrain from the sort of conduct that has always brought forth the dark skies in the past. I also have to be gentle enough with myself to realize that I am going to fail to hit the mark sometimes. I cannot afford to allow myself to wallow in self-contempt and self-pity. My faith is based on forgiveness and my testimony to that faith is to accept God's forgiveness, forgive myself, and try again.

Prayer
God, please strengthen my intestinal fortitude so that my character may continually be forged in a fashion that is pleasing to you. Amen

March 19

Thought for the day
He that will not apply new remedies must expect new evils,
for time is the greatest innovator.

Francis Bacon

Meditation
When our depression engulfs our lives, we have a very
difficult time believing that there are any remedies for our
condition. By its very nature, our depression tells us that our
situation is utterly hopeless. It tells us that it would be a
complete waste of time and effort to attempt to improve on
our condition. It tells us repeatedly that, even if there were
hope, we are worthless and do not deserve relief. What a
hideous condition we suffer from. We all need to continue
to take heart in the fact that these messages are nothing more
than the symptoms of this illness, and not our authentic
selves. We live in an age of constant medical miracles.
When we are out of the black hole, we need to be preparing
for our next bout. We need to look around our communities
and witness our fellow sufferers who are successfully
managing their lives in spite of their depression. When we
slip into a depression, we need to remember that the
condition will only be temporary and that time is truly the
greatest innovator. By preparing ourselves, we can get out
of the black hole much quicker than ever before.

Prayer
God thank you for the awareness that has allowed me to
successfully live with clinical depression. Thank you for the
belief system that I now have which tells me I do not have to
take my own life today. Amen

84

March 20

Thought for the day
Love, and do what you like.
St. Augustine

Meditation
When we are depressed, we are incapable of self-love. If we cannot love ourselves, we cannot authentically love another. Without love in our hearts, we lose our desire to live. And so the vicious cycle goes on. If you are treating your depression, accept your desire to overcome this illness as an outward sign of self-love. If you are struggling to make a beginning, please don't give up on yourself. You can find the peace that so many of us have found if only you will persevere till the end. What a freedom I have found by opening my mind to the idea that I can experience genuine love. What a freedom I have been blessed with, to believe that I can do anything that I desire, if I am willing to make the effort.

Prayer
God, please help all that suffer from depression to experience the self-love that is required to ask for help. Help us deny the messages that depression sends us and believe in your ability and desire to enter our hearts and minds. Amen

March 21

Thought for the day
Every new adjustment is a crisis in self-esteem.

Eric Hoffer

Meditation
I recall the day I was told that it was highly recommended I begin taking an anti-depressant medication. I felt like such a loser. I had to spend a considerable amount of time accepting and adjusting to my latest title, "clinically depressed". But out of that experience has developed some life-saving revelations, primarily the realization that it is much easier for me to stay clean and sober when I am treating my depression. The crisis in self-esteem, in regard to this matter, has since passed. I'm OK with it today.

Prayer
God thank you for seeing me through my scared and confused times by delivering me to the place of acceptance and understanding. Amen

March 22

Thought for the day
There is a secret person undamaged in every individual.

Paul Shepard

Meditation
When I consider a secret, undamaged self, which lives within me, I envision a cherub-like spirit resembling myself as a little boy. I imagine this spirit to be innocent and pure, unafraid and reliable. I see this child as constantly strong and extremely intelligent. He is unshaken by the chaos that my flesh surrounds him with. He has no concern with the flesh because he lives forever. He loves me so much, but he cannot be manipulated in the least by all my distractions. He is always cheering me on, yet is not discouraged by any of my failures. He remains steadfast and true. He is my authentic self.

Prayer
God, please help me embrace my authentic self and aspire to be all things that he represents. I know this is where the Holy Spirit resides within me. I want to feel the warmth of your love for me, yet I know my sin acts as a barrier and repels me away from your light. Please continue to shepherd me so I may find your truths. Amen

March 23

Thought for the day
Never look down to test the ground before taking your next
step; only he who keeps his eye fixed on the far horizon will
find his right road.

Dag Hammarskjold

Meditation
When I am depressed, I am consumed with negative
thoughts from the past as well as fears of the future. I will
negate all positive memories, only to dwell on my painful
mistakes. My present will be conceived as nothing short of
wretched, despite the lack of evidence to support my claim
of worthlessness. My ability to focus on the far horizon of
the future is limited by my lack of hope. But for the grace of
God, I no longer have to stare into the dark death of
depression. I am able to bring into mind, with the needed
force, the idea that I am experiencing the symptoms of a
treatable illness. Now I am able to lift my eyes to the sky
and ask for help.

Prayer
God, it was but a few years ago when I was unable to look
any person in the eye because I was so ashamed of myself. I
felt so phony and worthless that I just wanted to die. I began
to pray for your help, but felt that my prayers were falling on
deaf ears. I felt as though my sin had separated me from
your grace forever. I was too sick to realize that my prayers
would be answered, but in your time, not mine. Thank you.
Amen

March 24

Thought for the day
To achieve great things, we must live as though we were
never going to die.

Vauvenargues

Meditation
I suppose that the diametric expression would read
something like, *to achieve poor things, we must live as
though we were going to die today.* When we are consumed
with the gloom of our depression, we find ourselves
spending a considerable amount of time contemplating our
own death. We debate with ourselves whether we should
commit suicide and by what means. We consider methods of
self-destruction that might make our death appear to be
accidental. Perhaps we purposely become extremely
reckless, inviting death or hoping that somebody will notice
and intervene on our behalf. Whatever variety of self-
defeating thoughts we have, *and we have them all*, it is
important to note that we are not getting much of anything
else done. Our depression, if left untreated, robs us of our
lives. It takes away all of our hopes and dreams and replaces
them with thoughts of self-mutilation and death. Be honest
with yourself today. If you are experiencing the symptoms
of this illness, get help. If not for yourself, then for the
person you may help to save in the future.

Prayer
God, help us all continue to learn how to help ourselves so
that we may help others. Amen

March 25

Thought for the day
If you want something done right, get someone else to do it.
Marion Giacomini

Meditation
There are some things that I just cannot possibly do on my own. No matter how hard I try to manipulate, control, and exert my will, the desired results will not materialize. When I realize that my best efforts will not accomplish the task at hand, I become frustrated and disenchanted with the entire idea and abandon it. I lived my life for years trying unsuccessfully to bring about the changes of heart that I so desperately needed if I was ever going to know serenity and peace. The idea of somebody helping me was foreign. I always felt like I would owe you something if you aided me in any way. I believe my basic distrust of the human race fed my fear of being in debt to anybody. Also, somewhere along my journey through childhood, I picked up the message that I should feel ashamed of myself for needing help. What a wonderful gift I have today. I no longer have to be in absolute control. I can accept the fact that I am human and have some limitations. I can deal with the fact that I have some weaknesses that are somebody else's strength, and vise versa. It is a relief to no longer have to shoulder the burdens of the world, and allow someone else to "do it".

Prayer
God, help me be free from my fears, and allow me to peacefully participate in life. Show me when I need to stop pushing so hard, and just ask for help. Amen

March 26

Thought for the day
Many persons have a wrong idea of what constitutes true happiness. It is not attained through self-gratification but through fidelity to a worthy purpose.

Helen Keller

Meditation
Perhaps those of us who suffer from depression search more frantically for happiness than others. Maybe we do so because our lives depend on our ability to lift up out of the darkness of the black hole. The problem is that in our haste, we too readily look for happiness in places that it can never be found. Alcohol, drugs, sex, obsessive accumulation of wealth and power; all of these pursuits will never fill the void that is within our hearts. Millionaires die from all of the above quite frequently. True happiness must come from some other form or action. As it has been stated, happiness is not attained through self-gratification. True happiness can be found when helping others while expecting nothing in return. Often when I'm at my worst and know that I had better change my attitude quickly, I will look for somebody who needs a friend to talk with. It is important for me to listen to them and to be supportive, and to not discuss my self-perceived problems. I will undoubtedly walk away from my conversation feeling better about myself than if I had done all the talking.

Prayer
God, help us all find your path to true happiness. Help us learn that life is so much more rewarding when we are content to help others rather than always trying to help ourselves. Help us find the balance in life between taking care of ourselves in a healthy manner, and helping others. Amen

March 27

Thought for the day
What is hell? I maintain that it is the suffering of being unable to love.

Fyodor Dostoevsky

Meditation
Is it melodramatic to describe the black hole as hell? Is it hell for us to live when we are having yet another episode with depression? How does it feel to know that your best efforts to improve your outlook on life turn out to be nothing more than wishful thinking? Do you have the capacity to love or to feel loved when you are depressed? I know, from my personal experiences, that it is impossible for me to love when I am in the grip of depression. When I cannot think of one good reason to live another day, I am in a hell that only those of us who have experienced it can understand. That's why it is of the utmost importance that I have friends who also treat this illness. There have been many times when a member of my circle has pointed out to me that it appeared as though I might be slipping into a "funk". Today I will respect and respond to an observation such as this, and get into action doing what I need to do to help myself.

Prayer
God thank you for all of the love I have received during my entire recovery process. Thank you for the wonderful people you have put into my life. Without their support I don't know where I would be. Amen

March 28

Thought for the day
The strongest human instinct is to impart information, the second strongest is to resist it.

Kenneth Grahame

Meditation
I really enjoy talking with people today. I love to talk about recovery and to share my experience, strength, and hope with others. I achieve a great sense of worth when I am able to share some nuggets of wisdom with somebody, and they respond with a grateful smile. The truth is I do love to hear myself talk. I especially like it when I sound intelligent and people tell me that they enjoy listening to my message. From time to time, I can give some powerful advice, yet I will struggle on occasion, to heed my own words. If this is human instinct, I don't know why. I think it boils down to the fact that the difficult obstacles in life are easier to talk about than to actually solve. It is easy to talk about treating depression, but I know from my experience, that treating my depression requires effort and constant vigilance. Those words I need to never forget. My life truly does depend on it.

Prayer
God, I need your saving graces in so many ways. I often find myself giving good advice to somebody who has asked me for help, yet I know in my heart that I am not following my own words. Help me not just talk the talk but also walk the walk. Amen

March 29

Thought for the day
Make yourself necessary to somebody.
Ralph Waldo Emerson

Meditation
Untreated clinical depression will isolate you from people
and could kill you. It tells you that you are not necessary to
anybody and that the world would be a better place if you
were dead. Sound familiar? It is important that you force
yourself to be in contact with understanding people when
these thoughts occur. You need to be in touch with people
who will be honest with you and help you see where you are
necessary and to whom. If you live alone, perhaps you
befriend an elderly person who is lonely. Offer to put their
garbage on the curb on trash nights, or ask them to go to
dinner once a week. The point is that it is very important to
make a commitment to some person or group. You will be
surprised at what you get in return. It could save your life.

Prayer
God thank you for showing me how to help myself by
helping others. I know there have been some moments in the
past when I was less than secure in my recovery. Today, I
can look back and see that my commitments to others helped
motivate me to take care of myself by doing the next right
thing. Amen

March 30

Thought for the day
A man cannot be comfortable without his own approval.

Mark Twain

Meditation
Part of recovering from depression is to work on improving our self-esteem. When we are preoccupied with self-destructive and suicidal thoughts, our approval rating can be nowhere other than in the gutter. Most of us suffered from depression long before we ever realized it. During all those years that have passed us by, we have stumbled through the darkness feeling inferior and worthless. Changing our perception of ourselves does not occur overnight. I am resolved that I will have to guard against low self-esteem for the rest of my life. The difference in my life today is knowledge that I can change my attitudes and my perceptions anytime I want. Prior to recovery, I knew no other way.

Prayer
God, please continue to teach me and show me how to develop and maintain a healthy self-esteem. Protect me from self-defeating thoughts and activities so I may remain present and useful to others. Amen

March 31

Thought for the day
A blind man in a dark room – looking for a black hat which isn't there.

Lord Bowen

Meditation
How lost was I? I was a lost ball in tall grass. No, let's make that a lost green ball in tall grass. I was the blind man in a dark room – searching desperately for the black hat that was not there. I was the guy who was insanely pouring alcohol down his throat and free-basing cocaine to feel better. I was the guy who spent more energy devising ways to end his own life than it would have taken to ask for help. I was the guy who spent hours trying to find enough hose in the house to hook up to my exhaust pipe and run to the window of my car, but, because I'm such a perfectionist, it had to be the perfect diameter. It was important to look good, you know. I was the guy who was going to shoot himself in the head because he could not stop smoking "crack", only to give the gun to my crack dealer for more "crack". There is something comically tragic to be said about all this. I'm just grateful that I am able to look back on it today and find some humor in it. I know that at the time I was going through it, nobody was laughing. The good news that I share is that we do not have to live like that any more.

Prayer
God thank you for seeing me through the dark times. Please help those who still suffer from depression find the community of recovery that so many of us have been blessed with. Amen

April 1

Thought for the day
A man should not strive to eliminate his complexes, but to get into accord with them: they are legitimately what directs his conduct in the world.

Sigmund Freud

Meditation
Many of us have tried, to no avail, to overcome our *complexes* by denying their reality. We have attempted to be rid of the symptoms of depression by focusing on the world around us and pointing fingers at all that we perceived as disturbing. When the world does not come into our accord, we blame all that is involved for our depression. Then we debate suicide as a way to "show them" how badly their misconduct has hurt us. How insane is clinical depression? How unmanageable are our lives when we leave our depression unchecked and allow it to run amuck? Today we must face our shadows. We can no longer afford the lethal luxury of denial. We must accept our maladies and be honest with ourselves and all who may be placed in our lives to help us. Only then will we begin to know serenity and peace.

Prayer
God, help me continue to accept the reality of my existence. Help me understand that my maladies and shortcomings are mine to work on. Help me to understand that what I believe about myself and my illness will determine how I am able to treat it and heal. Amen

April 2

Thought for the day
Every April, God rewrites the Book of Genesis.

Unknown

Meditation
Life is the perpetual element of renewal. It is constantly renewing and reinventing itself. Whether we like it or not, we are part of this process. When we fight our need for change, when our soul cries out for a rebirth and we try to ignore it, we put ourselves at odds with the universe. We enter a stage of inner turmoil and unrest. The opportunities that we may rob ourselves of while resisting our natural need to change are countless and priceless. Fear is our greatest enemy. It tells us that any change we attempt to make will be for the worse. Our depression agrees and also reminds us that we do not deserve rebirth, but death. You do have the God given right to begin to change your life, starting today. If you are currently struggling to get out of the black hole, you do have the right to try something different today. You have the right to ask and receive help from somebody who truly understands and cares about you. You no longer have to cling to the insane notion that "this time it will be different". Graciously accept the help God has made available to you and renew yourself today.

Prayer
God, help me remember that I can begin my day over at anytime. Help me continue to be reborn and nurtured into a better human being. Show me that I do not have to stay stuck in my old ways any longer. Amen

April 3

Thought for the day
Give a man a fish and you feed him for a day. Teach a man
to fish and you feed him for a lifetime.

Chinese proverb

Meditation
When we are overwhelmed with depression, we often show
outward signs that we need and want help. Often these
expressions are misunderstood and only create bitterness and
resentment. On other occasions a friend or loved one may
attempt to "make it all better". Perhaps they succeed and we
find a temporary relief. What then happens during our next
episode? We look for the same response and outcome. If it
does not occur, it's now their fault. We become consumed
with the "if onlys", which will beget more depression. We
need to get our own help. We need to learn to fish so that we
may be fed for a lifetime. It is our responsibility to get all
the help and information that we need to arrest the symptoms
of this illness.

Prayer
God, today I am responsible for my recovery. It is my job to
see to it that I am taking care of myself. Help me never
scapegoat another person for how I feel. By blaming others
and not helping myself, I will not get better. I will stay
stuck. Thank you for the courage and strength to go forward
resolved to the fact that I must take care of myself. Amen

April 4

Thought for the day
I have never seen a greater monster or miracle in the world than myself.

Montaigne

Meditation
It is an absolute miracle that I am alive and sober today. I had lost all hope that I would ever achieve sobriety, let alone find a joyful, productive way of life. I frequently have to force myself to relax because I am still nervous about the bottom falling out and my life returning to hell. I know that treating my depression has made my sobriety possible. Prior to recovery, I was filled with so much rage that I actually felt like I was under demonic influence. I wanted to devour anybody who hurt me and then kill myself. I cannot imagine returning to that pain and insanity. I know it all still awaits me. If I do not treat my depression, I am jeopardizing the welfare of my family and my life. It is that real today.

Prayer
God thank you for the miracle of my life today. I fear returning to the "monster" and the life I once lived. I want to remain in your pocket of grace. Please protect me from allowing my spiritual condition to decay to the point of collapse. Teach me to do your will, not mine. Amen

April 5

Thought for the day
We judge ourselves by our motives and others by their actions.   **Dwight Morrow**

Meditation
How difficult has it been for our loved ones to live with us while we were suffering from depression? Most likely they made every attempt to help us change our mood... to make us happy. As we responded negatively to their actions, they have been left feeling frustrated and angry. We in turn are in our own hell because we cannot even begin to explain why we feel the way we do. I usually would put the blame directly on my family's actions, the very actions that were designed to help me. As my condition worsened, I would become angry with myself because I could see the pain and distress I was causing my family. This of course only led to more depression. And so the cycle goes. Does untreated depression destroy families? You bet it does. Does it affect the lives of innocent children? Absolutely! The first thing I had to work on once I began my recovery process was to stop blaming my family for how I felt. Today, when I am depressed, I let them know that I feel depressed and that it is not their fault. I let them know that it is something for me to work through and that everything will be fine. As a result of this new approach, they feel more secure, which in turn helps me to feel better.

Prayer
God, help me continue to treat my depression as an illness and not the result of somebody else's actions. Help me be honest and open about how I am feeling, and share that information with my family and friends. Help them understand that clinical depression is a treatable illness, and not their fault. Amen

April 6

Thought for the day
Every man shall bear his own burden.
Galatians 6:5

Meditation
I can be very grateful about all the burdens I don't have today. I used to cry "why me?" Today I can respond, " why not me?" The world is full of people who are suffering. I believe that there still are people on this planet who have never seen water come out of a faucet...poor folks who do not have enough to eat or adequate shelter. People who cannot walk or see. Children who are afflicted with deadly infections and viruses...with no means to obtain the available medical attention that we enjoy. The list goes on. If I am honest with myself about my burdens, I must admit that my life could be much worse. Sometimes when I am depressed, I will take a look at the world that I live in and find something that I am grateful I don't have to deal with. It helps me to lighten my burden and take care of myself. I also have to remember that every man shall bear his own burdens...that the people who appear so happy and perfect really are human beings who have their own problems to contend with. I have befriended such people over the years, and after closer examination, I have concluded that I wouldn't want to trade places with them. Today, I'll be OK being me.

Prayer
God, today I will accept my burdens as my problems to overcome. I will remember that my life could be much worse. I will work toward being grateful for all that I have. Amen

April 7

Thought for the day
Nothing great is created suddenly, any more than a bunch of
grapes or a fig. If you tell me that you desire a fig, I answer
you that there must be time. Let it first blossom, then bear
fruit, then ripen.

Epictetus

Meditation
There has been nothing instant about my recovery. At times
it has seemed pitifully slow, if not stuck. Sometimes it has
felt as if I was racing in reverse. I have learned to be patient
with my process. That is not to say that I'm happy about the
turnaround time. I still can become very impatient. I have
grown to expect instant gratification in my life.
Consequently, I have stood clear of anything that would
require much staying power on my part. I am always
looking for conclusions. I have to continue to learn how to
enjoy the process. That is what is important in my life today
because my recovery is ongoing and must continue to renew
itself, bringing forth-new fruit for seasons to come.

Prayer
God, help me understand that there are no quick fixes for my
life today. I must continue to learn patience and trust the
process. I must draw upon the history of my success and
bear witness to the fact that all has worked out well, in your
speed. Amen

April 8

Thought for the day
The days come and go like muffled and veiled figures sent from a distant friendly party, but they say nothing, and if we do not use the gifts they bring, they carry them as silently away.

Ralph Waldo Emerson

Meditation
Today is the first day of the rest of our lives, and what we make of it is entirely up to us. If we spend the rest of today trying to discover what is wrong with it, inevitably we will find nothing but fault. Likewise, if we search for all that is right, we will find good. It is when I choose to be open-minded and optimistic, that I begin to notice all the wonderful things that life has to offer me. It is when I believe in myself, that I can become excited about today. When I spend the better part of my day making funeral arrangements, the gifts that this day has to offer sweep right past me. I must be present in the moment to seize the moment. It is not easy to stay that focused, but I have tasted life in the moment and it is where I want to be.

Prayer
God, help me seize the moments of my life and live in the now. Help me become more at ease with myself. Help me know peace. Amen

April 9

Thought for the day
How to make God laugh. Tell him your future plans.

Woody Allen

Meditation
I am a recovering person. I am also a therapist and a caretaker. I am also a husband and a parent. I also suffer from bouts of depression. These are all qualifiers to let you know that I truly understand God's sense of humor. Growing up in a dysfunctional family, I learned that I was supposed to be in total control of my life and that of the people I cared about. God must have had many laughs while watching my relentless efforts to achieve such an impossible goal. When I came into recovery, I began to understand that control in most forms was merely an illusion. I attempted to control my children with all the justification and rationalizing I could...only to finally understand it was their lives not mine. I have learned that the curse put on me by my parents is now passed on to my children. You see...my parents' efforts to control me also failed. I am reminded on a daily basis at work how much energy is wasted on planning outcomes. I make a strategic plan to use with my patients' in-group. It is a great plan. I start out with the great plan, and I always end up somewhere else. Thank God I have learned to be an instrument...otherwise God would laugh alone.

Prayer
God, please allow me to continue to plan with the ability to let go of the outcome for others and myself. Give me the courage and strength to ask for your help and the help of others throughout the day so that I may accept life on life's terms. Amen

April 10

Thought for the day
FEAR – False Evidence Appearing Real
Unknown

Meditation
I can remember when FEAR ruled my world and kept me concealed in a cloak of depression. I could not come out because of the overwhelming fear I had. The insanity of this is related to the fact that when I am experiencing FEAR, it appears to be very real. I now have a support system in place for these occasions. I cannot wait until I need the support. If I wait to ask for the support when I need it, it is too late. I have to set up my support system before FEAR hits so that they are there and ready to help me get through the FEAR. Getting through the FEAR means I need to find the evidence of what is real. When that dark cloud is hovering overhead, I am unable to see FEAR for what it really is without the help of others.

Prayer
God, am I truly humble enough to know that I cannot make it through my bouts of depression without your help and the help of others? Please allow me to surrender my belief that I can do this alone. Amen

April 11

Thought for the day
Once a man would spend a week patiently waiting if he missed a stagecoach, but now he rages if he misses the first section of a revolving door.

Simeon Strunsky

Meditation
We live in an era of instant gratification. Everything has to be quick. Quick service, quick results, with the least amount of effort required. That is what we have come to think of as good. Our media reinforces this idea of "fast relief", but sometimes it just does not work. There isn't always a quick cure. Worse yet, sometimes things don't quite work as advertised. When it comes to treating our depression, we must learn patience. If we are placed on anti-depressants, we may have to switch medications numerous times until we find the one or combination that best works for us. We must accept that we might find something that works for a period of time, but may soon fade, forcing us to ask for help yet one more time. And most importantly, we may have to accept the fact that we might have to treat our depression, one day at a time, for the rest of our lives.

Prayer
God thank you for your blessing of patience and acceptance. Help me remember that there are no quick fixes when it comes to my recovery. It's a daily reprieve that I have been granted. Thank you. Amen

April 12

Thought for the day
…Go toward all the life there is with all the courage you can find and all the belief you can muster. Be brave, be true, stand. All the rest is darkness.

Stephen King

Meditation
Sometimes courage and faith seem like concepts from an alien world. It would be so much easier to hide in the darkness, perhaps picking up the gun or the pills and making it all permanent. But I have friends and family…and most of all myself, to whom I must be true. So I get on my knees and I pray for courage. And if I have faith, I find that very soon I can go forward, into the light and into the future. I can be brave and stand with my fellow sufferers. Together, we can escape the darkness.

Prayer
God, help me remember that you are always present in my life, even when I feel as though you are not. Help me remember that with a little faith and a little bravery, I can make it through anything. Amen

April 13

Thought for the day
I mean by this sacrament an outward and visible sign of an
inward and spiritual grace.

Book of Common Prayer

Meditation
The purpose of my writing these meditations is two-fold.
First, it is my sincerest desire that I may inspire and move
some lost soul's heart toward God and recovery. Second is
to give all the glory to my God. I count each day of my life,
each day sober, each day without a suicidal thought as a
testimony of God's everlasting saving grace. If one person
and his or her family can be spared the agony of a suicide,
then let that be my outward sign of my inward desire to help
in some small way. But let the glory be for the Great Spirit,
for without, I surely would have already perished.

Prayer
God, I need your strength in my life always. It is by your
saving grace that I live yet another day to serve you. Please
free me from my sins and temptations so that I may be more
consistently available to do your work. Amen

April 14

Thought for the day
We must indeed all hang together, or most assuredly we shall all hang separately.

Benjamin Franklin

Meditation
Much can be said about the accomplishments of community. One of the greatest community movements that has occurred this century is that of the fellowship of Alcoholics Anonymous. The success rate of alcoholics achieving continuous sobriety prior to the advent of AA in 1935 was precarious at best. Today, millions of men, women, and even children are maintaining sobriety as a result of practicing the program's principles and participating in the fellowship. I can attest to the fact that the community of recovering depression sufferers has indeed saved my life. But these people didn't just show up at my door one day. I had to seek them out. I had to ask them for their phone numbers. I had to say, " I need help".

Prayer
God, please direct me so that I never isolate myself from you or my friends again. Help me remember how important it is for me to participate in my recovery...to be available for others whenever they may call upon me for help. Amen

April 15

Thought for the day
There is nothing noble about being superior to some other man. The true nobility is in being superior to your previous self.

Hindu proverb

Meditation
When we are in the grips of depression and we feel like we cannot go on, there remains in us, deep within our souls, a burning instinct to survive. If this were not true, we all would have taken our own lives long ago. So we carry on for years, contemplating our own demise, feeling like cowards and failures because we can't even kill ourselves right. Then, by the grace of God, we get help. We begin to treat our illness, using a multitude of resources, and we find relief. For some of us, the fight is more difficult than for others. We may find ourselves making comparisons to others, trying in vain to measure up. If we calculate that we do not exceed the standard we have chosen, we conclude that we are doomed to failure. But if our yardstick is our previous self, how much have we grown? We can know our own true nobility when we stop trying to be superior to others, and only compare ourselves to our previous self.

Prayer
God, please teach me how to keep the focus on myself. Help me to accept myself for what I am, and show me how to grow and respond to my growth in a positive, healthy way. Amen

April 16

From error to error one discovers the entire truth.

Sigmund Freud

Meditation
There was a time in my life, not so long ago, that I walked amid the shattered pieces of all my hopes and dreams. My body felt worn and tattered, and I just wanted to end it all. How I ever mustered the will to live, I may never know. My errors in the past taught me that I needed help. My wounds, left by my own transgressions, ran deep...wounds that have since healed but have left visible scars. If I press on them, they will trigger pain, so I try to protect them the best I can. Today, as I turn from my erroneous ways in search of the truth, I am able to begin mending what was damaged in my wake of sickness and self-will.

Prayer
God, help me learn the healing messages that are contained within my errors. Help me understand that through my tribulations, I have become the person that I am today. Amen

April 17

Thought for the day
Blessed are they who heal us of self-despisings. Of all services which can be done to man, I know of none more precious.

William Hale White

Meditation
Feeling less-than, worthless, evil, unloving, etc., was so ingrained into my self-perception that I continuously have to make a conscious effort not to fall back into my old way of viewing myself. It has taken the loving support of many wonderful people for me to become willing to consider that just maybe I was being a little hard on myself. I once attended a five-day family program for the purpose of improving my self-esteem. I revealed some of my deepest pains to my group. Although I felt that I should have been brought to tears as I opened up, it did not occur. When I cried is when I was finished telling my story and the therapist started to say nice things about me. It was so difficult for me to hear these things, even more difficult to accept them as truths. As the five days came to an end, we said our good byes. The therapists handed all of us little cardboard signs that said, "I am important". I really felt like I was. Thank God for the people who are out there making a difference. If you do not have people like that in your life, then you must find them now. You deserve it because you are important too!

Prayer
God thank you for all the loving, caring people that you have put in my life. Help me remember that it is now my responsibility to be a loving, caring person for somebody else. Amen

April 18

Thought for the day
Compassion for myself is the most powerful healer of them all.

Theodore Isaac Rubin

Meditation
Compassion for yourself means that you do deserve recovery. It means that you can forgive yourself for past transgressions. It means that it is OK to ask for help. It allows you to have limitations and to set boundaries. When you are depressed, compassion for yourself means not listening to the self-defeating thoughts that are racing through your mind. It means separating yourself from the illness and then taking the necessary steps to begin healing. It says that you do deserve relationships that are based on intimacy and trust. Compassion for yourself means that you are loving and loveable. And finally, compassion for yourself says that God loves you exactly at this moment, exactly as you are.

Prayer
God, please continue to teach me how to have compassion for myself. Help me to know your peace. Amen

April 19

Thought for the day
If you really do put a small value upon yourself, rest assured that the world will not raise your price.

Unknown

Meditation
How does it feel when a loved one, after unsuccessfully attempting to raise your spirits, becomes frustrated and shakes their head with disgust and walks away? When you see their complete deflation of hope, what goes through your mind? I would usually respond by concluding that I was, in fact, a worthless piece of dung, and that I would be doing the world a favor if I were to just drop dead. Is it our loved one's responsibility that we feel like that? Absolutely not! They meant well. Perhaps they don't know the first thing about clinical depression. Why should they? We have not yet told them that they didn't cause it and they can't cure it. And so the cycle continues. We continue to allow ourselves to remain untreated and our depression continues to rob us of our self-worth. We remain in our own filth while life passes us by. How tragic is this illness? Is it real? Every time I hear of a suicide I know that untreated depression took another life. If you need help today, get it. If you don't need help today, find somebody who does and help them out. One day they may save your life.

Prayer
God, depression robs me of my self-worth. Help me continue my recovery and improve how I feel about "me" today. Show me my true importance and value to mankind by allowing me to help somebody else. Amen

April 20

Thought for the day
Anything you're good at contributes to happiness.

Bertrand Russell

Meditation
Some days it is very difficult for me to feel like I am good at much of anything. Yet, I have to remember that we all have been blessed with certain gifts, and even though I may not be at the top of my game, I still can make a difference and contribute to happiness. It is extremely easy for me to be helpful and useful when I feel grand. I imagine that I am not unique in that regard. The true test of my character lies in my ability to display what I am good at and to contribute to happiness when I am feeling less than worthy. My recovery tells me that I can and must try to do this even when it does not feel right. My faith tells me that I must trust in my God and be ready to help others regardless of where I may be emotionally. I have to continue to recall that whenever I have made an attempt to help somebody without any expectations, I have always experienced a sense of joy and usefulness. I also have to look at the fact that, on many occasions, by being in a certain space or frame of mind, I was able to better serve the person that, out of the blue, appeared in my life. I can no longer deny the rhythm of the Great Spirit of Life.

Prayer
God thank you for the many blessings and gifts you have given me. Help me use my gifts to help others in a way that you find pleasing. Amen

April 21

Thought for the day
I'm a slow walker, but I never walk back.

Abraham Lincoln

Meditation
I like the idea of never walking back. I think it is very important to remember where we came from so that we may continue to recognize where we are headed. Other than that, it can be very dangerous for us to wallow in the past. Today is the day that God has made...and what you choose to do with the rest of this day is entirely up to you. Are you going to try to fix your life in one day? Are you going to attempt to jam twenty-four months of recovery into twenty-four hours? I am capable of attempting both. My aim is a little different today. I'll be the slow walker. I'll be the slow walker if that will result in steady growth. My experience has already taught me that there are no quick fixes here. My recovery truly is one day at a time for the rest of my life. Sometimes I get impatient; I want to feel great right now and forevermore. I want things to be perfect. Unfortunately, I'm the guy defining perfection and my definition of perfect only seems to exist in fairytales. So, on occasion, I need to slow way down. I need to meditate on being a slow walker, making steady progress, one day at a time. This will require diligence and practice. Whoever promised us that it would be easy, anyhow?

Prayer
God, today I ask for the courage and strength to pursue steady growth. Please guide me away from chasing the dreams of quick fixes. Help me remember that the true reward lies in diligence and practice. Amen

April 22

Thought for the day
We promise according to our hopes, and perform according to our fears.

La Rochefoucauld

Meditation
So often when we are in the early stages of depression, we start to promise ourselves that, if we take certain actions, we will feel better. We try to brush off the symptoms as fatigue, anger, loneliness etc., and promise ourselves that getting some rest, getting over our anger, or finding somebody to be with, will relieve us of our pain. In and of themselves, all these solutions do have their merit. The problem lies in the central fact that these feelings may be the result of our illness, and unless we treat the illness, the symptoms may not go away. We are deceiving ourselves when our hopes are not based in reality. We can no more hope that our "blues" dissipate when we are in the grips of clinical depression, than we can hope our coughing away when we suffer from pneumonia. My fears, once they become overwhelming, have always motivated me into action. In the past, those actions were inappropriate. Today I have a healthy fear of my depression. That fear motivates me to perform certain tasks so that I may quickly get my depression under control and resume my life.

Prayer
God, help me be honest with myself today. Help me remember that wishful thinking is not going to get me very far in regard to treating my depression. It is appropriate action on my part that is required. Please continue to supply me with the courage and strength that I need. Amen

April 23

Thought for the day
Anxiety is fear of one's self.
Wilhelm Stekel

Meditation
I have lived my entire life running from the shadows cast by my clouds of impending doom. Riddled with fear, I have anxiously awaited the catastrophes of my life to unfold. At times, the suspense of the conclusion could be more than I could bear, so I would exercise whatever actions were necessary to bring about my self-defeating, self-fulfilling prophecy. How much of a role untreated clinical depression played in this insanity is open for debate. I can say with certainty that there were other elements to blame, but with the same certainty, I can confirm that since my recovery, I am acutely aware of the fact that living beneath the shadows of impending doom is a self-perceived hell and not the reality of life. And so, with this proclamation, I carry on. I live with the knowledge that faith in God, and the process called life, will overcome my fear. Now, I must apply this awareness as a magnifying glass to permeate the light of life, through the clouds of impending doom, into my heart.

Prayer
God, please continue to teach me how to live within the reality of life, and not under the shadows of my self-perceived impending doom. Help me apply to my daily living, the awareness and inspiration that you have provided me. Amen

April 24

Thought for the day
Neither do men light a candle and put it under a bushel, but on a candlestick; and it giveth light unto all that are in the house.

Matthew 5:15

Meditation
What must we do with our light of recovery? How should we disburse the wisdom that we have been blessed with? Should we hold it unto ourselves? Should we illuminate a room that is already lit? Or should we find the darkness and become a beacon of light for all those who are lost in the blackness of depression? How do we maintain our light? Who replenishes it if it should become dim? By the grace of God, I am learning that the fuel for my fire is obtained by helping others. It is also by the same grace that I have grown to accept that when I am lost in the darkness, I need another's light to find my way clear. Without your light placed on a candlestick, I will wander aimlessly in the darkness of the black hole. If you are presently in the darkness, walk toward the light. If today, you are the light, let it shine!

Prayer
God, please show me how to best illuminate your paths to recovery from clinical depression. Help me accept the awesome responsibility that I have to help others. Let me in turn seek the light of other recovering people when I am in the dark. Amen

April 25

Thought for the day
Change is not made without inconvenience, even from worse
to better.   **Richard Hooker**

Meditation
Breaking familiar patterns of behavior is difficult. Even if
the change will be for our betterment, it is natural to resist
any break from what we might consider normal. There is a
sense of security in habit, whether the habit is healthy or not.
The security is achieved by knowing the outcome that will
occur as a result of repeating the same process. How does
this behavior relate to treating depression? First, I have to
admit that there is an element of control involved when I am
having a bout with depression. When I am depressed, the
people around me react in a fairly predictable fashion. I
guess the analogy would be "walking on eggshells", and in a
really sick way, I can achieve a sense of power from that
experience. I am certain if you are honest with yourself, you
may recall at least one time when you attempted to
manipulate another person's behavior with your depression.
When we are depressed, we desperately need approval. If
we can get other people to respond to us in this fashion, we
sometimes are able to wrench some self-worth out of the
experience. Part of our recovery is giving up the game of
manipulation and control. It's about being honest, and
letting our family and friends off the hook.

Prayer
God, empower me to make the right changes in my life
today. Help me be honest with myself regarding the true
nature of my condition. When I am down, let me not try to
manipulate and control others behaviors in an attempt to feel
better. Show me your direction to sane living, one day at a
time. Amen

April 26

Thought for the day
Here I stand. I can do no other. God help me. Amen
Martin Luther

Meditation
I have spent much of my life feeling like a phony. I have carried with me the constant companion of inadequacy and have tried desperately to compensate for my inadequacies by faking my way through life. As a result, I developed a mental outlook that was clouded with illusions, and a perception of reality that was distorted. My recovery has been a painful exploration into my soul to save my authentic self. As I unearthed enough dishonesty, I began to uncover me. With the help of some wonderful people, I was pulled out from the quicksand of inadequacy and set firmly on healthy ground. At that moment I stood again. I could do no other because I had learned that my old way of thinking did not work. Yet, I knew no other way. My friends said "pray". I prayed, "God please help me". God answered by allowing me to see all the help that surrounded me. He said, "Faith without works is dead - now it is time to get to work". I did.

Prayer
Here I stand. I can do no other. God help me. Amen

April 27

Thought for the day
A cynic can chill and dishearten with a single word.
Ralph Waldo Emerson

Meditation
When we are depressed, we can chill and dishearten even the happiest of times. We are so engulfed in the darkness that we are unable to see the light of life. Essentially, we really don't have anything good to say about anything. I was always acutely aware of how miserably I responded to my family when I was dying in the black hole. It was easy for me to hate myself for my words and deeds. I couldn't understand why I was such an uncooperative, miserable, mean person. Of course initially, I would blame the people in my life for how I felt. They would instinctively lash out and shake my misplaced burden off their shoulders back onto mine. I would respond with a conclusion that I now had all the evidence I needed to no longer stay my execution, and carry out my death plan. How difficult is it for our family and friends, when we leave our depression untreated? This illness kills people. It spiritually kills all those who love us. Let us not forget that it is our responsibility to get the help we need so that we can start enjoying life again, and in the process, share our new found joy with those people who have waited for years to see us smile again.

Prayer
God, this illness called depression has destroyed so many lives. Lives of husbands, wives, and children have been turned upside down by the insanity of the clinically depressed. Give us all the strength to unite and raise public awareness of this killer to a new level so that the lives of countless numbers of people can be saved. Amen

April 28

Thought for the day
Human life consists in mutual service. No grief, pain,
misfortune, or "broken heart" is excuse for cutting off one's
life while any power of service remains. But when all
usefulness is over, when one is assured of an unavoidable
and imminent death, it is the simplest of human rights to
choose a quick and easy death in place of a slow and horrible
one.

Suicide note, **Charlotte Perkins Gilman**

Meditation
I initially felt uncomfortable presenting a suicide note to my
fellow depression sufferers. Then I realized that most of us
have already written such a note at one time or another, and
some of us, myself included, have "come to" after a failed
attempt to take our own life, only to read our note again. On
my list of depressing moments, I would say that the
"morning after" read of the pathetic note I scribed the night
before, tops the list. That being said, I want to share some
observations that I made after reading the suicide note above.
At first, it made sense to me. Of course it did. I suffer from
depression. But upon closer examination, I began to
discover cracks in the philosophy contained within. The
error in thinking occurred when Charlotte wrote, *but when
all usefulness is over...*my response is, according to whom?
I am certain that she felt that there was no usefulness left in
her being. I am just as certain that she suffered from
depression and died because of it. We all are familiar with
the symptoms. The challenge we are faced with today is to
be rigorously honest about our ability to be useful. My
recovery has taught me that if I can still pick up litter off the
street, I am useful. If I can still read a book to a child, I am
useful.

If I can share my feelings about depression with another person, I am useful. If I can still pray to God, I am useful.

Prayer
God, my depression can rob me of all feelings of usefulness. It tells me I have nothing worthwhile to contribute to society. When I am in this frame of mind, please allow me the inspiration to realize that these feelings are not fact. Amen

April 29

Thought for the day
A man's dying is more the survivors' affair than his own.

Thomas Mann

Meditation
When we are suffering from depression, it can be very difficult for us to consider the feelings of others. Our thought processes are so self-defeating that when we do think of others, we rationalize that they do not really give a damn whether we breathe another moment or not. We think that we will not really be missed by anybody and that our family would be much better off if we were to just die. It is very important that when we are on stable ground we examine the validity of this sort of thinking. We are all going to know a physical death. There are three hundred sixty-five days in a year and one of those days is ours to die on. My faith in the existence of a God provokes me to abandon the idea that taking my own life would ever be natural and in accordance with God's will for me. Beyond that, it would be the most selfish, self-centered act I could ever perform…and what about my survivors? I can say with a clear conscience that the vision of my two sons looking into my casket as a result of taking my own life has provided me, at times, with sufficient enough distraction not to pull the trigger. But there have been times in my life when not even my love for my children prevented me from making a valid attempt at my life. So from this I have learned to prepare myself for my next bout with depression. I have learned that during my up times, I must cross-examine the lies that this illness will attempt to use to kill me. I must be honest with myself regarding the excruciating pain my suicide would cause others. Whether you believe it or not, yours would too.

126

Prayer

God, when I am depressed, I consider the hideous act of suicide as a way out. I struggle to believe anybody would be hurt by this action. Help me see through these lies and understand these feelings are a symptom of an illness and not my authentic self. Amen

April 30

Thought for the day
God will not look you over for medals, degrees or diplomas,
but for scars!

Elbert Hubbard

Meditation
During the course of my life, I have acquired my fair share
of physical and mental scars...scars that are a direct result of
untreated depression. I am not alone. Many of us have, or
know friends who have the slashing scars that remain after
we attempt to slit our wrists. Others have collapsed veins
and damaged skin from intravenous drug use and/or scars on
their internal organs from alcohol abuse. But the scars that
run the deepest are emotional scars. Today, my scars are a
daily reminder of where I came from and how close I came
to ending my life. By all accounts I should be dead. They
also serve to remind me of the valiant fight I have made to
get where I am at today. We should all feel a sense of heroic
victory when we survive yet another trip to the black hole. It
is good for all of us to learn how to be proud of our recovery.
To the outside world, our joy may not be understood. But
we know what it's like to suffer from this illness. God
knows too!

Prayer
God, my illness has left many scars on my body, some
external, many more, internal. Help me continue to gain
wisdom from the experiences that have left their marks in
my life so I may not repeat old patterns of self-destructive
behavior. Amen

May 1

Thought for the day
Unto whomsoever much is given, of him shall much be required.   **Luke 12:48**

Meditation
Today we have been blessed with the opportunity to continue our recovery from depression and to help others. Despite the trials and tribulations we may encounter today, we must always draw from the well of hope the belief that today is worth fighting for. Every human being has been given a calling of sorts. Some, blinded by fear and self-will, live their entire life without ever discovering what it is that they are to be "doing". I consider it a blessing that I am alive and sober today. Some days I become overcome with grief and fear. Nothing feels right. I become very frustrated with myself because my plans are not unfolding the way I desire. It is when I reach the point of giving up that I am usually inspired to consider the fact that I am already living on borrowed time. My plans really are not that important. I already have all I need. Anything else would just be icing on the cake. We all like icing, but we know we can live without it. So today we must consider the awesome gift we have been given... recovery from an illness that will kill people today. We also must focus, not so much on our daily living problems, but on what is required of us. Today our number one requirement is to help each other heal from the wounds of depression.

Prayer
God thank you for the precious gift of recovery. I have been given my life back as a result of the wonderful people you have put in my life. Help me remember that if I want to keep this precious gift, I must always be ready to share it with others. Amen

May 2

Thought for the day
I expect to pass though this world but once. Any good therefore that I can do, or any kindness that I can show to my fellow-creature, let me do it now. Let me not defer or neglect it, for I shall not pass this way again.

Attributed to **Stephen Grellet**

Meditation
Years ago, I met a very wise and virtuous man who had a plan for simple daily living. He told me that each day he makes certain that he performs at least one random act of kindness. He added that it was very important that the act remain anonymous. He was one of the happiest, calmest, people I have ever encountered. Unfortunately, for those of us who suffer from untreated depression, this way of living seems impossible. Our depression has robbed us of so much. The joys of a simple and serene life are ripped from our souls, only to be replaced by a life consumed with constant thoughts of self-contempt and self-mutilation. Do you deserve a better life today? Should you be able to experience the joys of giving without needing anything in return? You better believe you do! Today, if your depression is in remission, go help somebody by performing a random act of kindness. If you are depressed, call out for help so that somebody else may enjoy giving. See, by reaching out for help, you are also helping somebody else.

Prayer
God, please don't allow me to waste any more of my life on destructive ideas. Grant me the wisdom and the vision to see where I can do good. Amen

May 3

Thought for the day
If a friend is in trouble, don't annoy him by asking if there is anything you can do. Think up something appropriate and do it.

Edgar Watson Howe

Meditation
Part of my recovery process is to spend time with other people who suffer from this illness. We all are aware that when we are slipping toward the black hole, we are usually the last to know. So we look after one another. These are by far the purest friendships I have ever encountered. They are one of the greatest fringe benefits of no longer trying to do this on my own. Beyond that, when a friend notices that I am starting to exhibit the symptoms of this illness, they never ask me if there is anything that they can do. They already know what my reply will be. No! Why would I want any help? I'm depressed and don't think I deserve help. We are all too familiar with the cycle. What I get from my friends is sound direction. They tell me to call my doctor immediately. They tell me that they will call me to see if I called my doctor. They tell me that if I do not call my doctor, they will come and get me and take me to the hospital. They will make me make a commitment to get together with them in the very near future. They will call other people in my circle of support and tell them that I am having another bout. Those people will start calling me. All these people will help me through the darkness and see to it that I arrive safely on the shores of the light. Their direction saves me from weeks or months of unnecessary suffering. It could be argued that their efforts possibly save my life. This is the way it works my friend. If you do not have people like this in your life. Find them! We are everywhere.

Prayer
God thank you for my friends in recovery. It is their understanding of this illness that allows them the wisdom to know how to truly help me when I am suffering. I pray for the people that are lost right now, who are suffering and do not know where to turn. Please help them find their way toward the healing that they deserve. Amen

May 4

Thought for the day
Calmness is always Godlike.

Ralph Waldo Emerson

Meditation
People who do not suffer from depression cannot understand the excruciating pain and the devilish turmoil that we experience when we are in the black hole of despair. They look upon us with that confused "you are crazy" look, which only begets more depression. As we slip deeper into the darkness of our depression, we may become enraged and venomous. We say incredibly evil things to the people that we love. Perhaps they tell us that we are over-reacting to the event that we are blaming for our ill feelings. They tell us we need to relax. We flip out because they do not understand. Neither do we. Calmness is not achievable at this time. The ability to have faith in God is also absent. We need help. Accepting the fact that all of the above are symptoms of an illness and not our authentic selves is the first major step toward recovery and the Godlike calmness that we have desperately been searching for. We must remember to let our families off the hook. It's not their fault. They may have hurt us terribly in the past, but nothing that they have done adds up to taking our own life. If your husband or wife has abandoned you, please carry on. You have no idea what God has in store for you. Get the help you deserve. Get healthy. Do not quit before the miracle happens. Your miracle is awaiting you.

Prayer
God, help me know your calmness. Show me how to relax and live with serenity and peace. Allow me the faith to believe that despite the hurt I may be experiencing, it will get better. Amen

133

May 5

Thought for the day
When one door of happiness closes, another opens; but often we look so long at the closed door that we do not see the one which has been opened for us.

Helen Keller

Meditation
We all experience periods of sadness and grief in our life. Lost relationships, lost loved ones, lost jobs, etc... they have all caused us to experience feelings of depression, and so they should. In recovery, I have learned that it is appropriate for me to mourn these losses for a period of time. But at some point I must accept the circumstances as reality by allowing the door to close on my loss, and allowing myself to look for open doors of opportunity elsewhere. This process is normal and healthy. But when I am clinically depressed, all doors are slammed shut right in my face and dead-bolted. The only doors that I can find to open are the closet doors that are filled with all my skeletons and painful memories. As I stand lost in the darkness of the dingy hallway filled with all these locked doors, I discover a murky, decaying wooden window to escape from. I run toward it, considering as I run, whether I should just throw myself through it and plunge to my catastrophic end. There seems to be no way out. But then, by the grace of God, I notice an old, vandalized pay phone hanging in the far corner of my hell. I am certain that it must be out of order. I know that even if it docs work, nobody is going to come help me out. Yet I am compelled to try. I pick up the phone and begin to dial for help. At that moment, I hear the sound of all the dead bolts sliding back into their housings. I look, and there is light squeezing out from underneath the doors. Suddenly, the doors gently begin to open and help arrives. Now I am able, once again, to see the doors of happiness.

Prayer

God, help me never to give up hope in my ability to renew myself. Help me understand that sadness over a loss is to be expected. Allow me to grieve my losses properly and then to shut the door on them, only to find the next door of opportunity open. Amen

May 6

Thought for the day
Being entirely honest with oneself is a good exercise.
Sigmund Freud

Meditation
It is not easy for me to be entirely honest at all times. In fact it is difficult for me to be entirely honest some of the time. The person that I have the most trouble being honest with is "me". I have an incredible ability to rationalize the most insane notions into something that comes close to resembling sound thinking. A large part of my recovery has been unearthing the truth from beneath the layers of rationalization that I have accumulated over the years. It is very good exercise for me. But, not unlike physical exercise, it is sometimes difficult for me to find the motivation to get started. Even more difficult is sustaining some sort of training schedule that is frequent enough to produce favorable results. And of course pain and effort are involved. We who suffer from depression sometimes have to fight an uphill battle. If we are depressed, we say to ourselves, "what's the use anyhow?" Yet, that is probably the most important time to become rigorously honest regarding the illness of depression and the symptoms that we may be exhibiting. It is very important that I continue to pursue complete honesty. I will never be perfect at it, but I'll be a much better person for trying.

Prayer
God, today allow me to be honest with myself. Grant me the courage to remove the years of rationalization from my thoughts, and uncover the entire truths about my motives and desires. Amen

May 7

Thought for the day
All men by nature desire to know.
Aristotle

Meditation
Throughout my life, my persistent pessimism and emotional awkwardness have left me searching for the knowledge of why I suffer from feelings that never quite seem appropriate for the moment. Being the analytical person that I am, I have spent countless hours rehashing happenings in my mind, trying to discover enough evidence to support my argument for discontent or over-reacting. The flames of depression only fan my obsession to know that much more. I must have reasonable justification for how I feel or else I perceive that I am losing my mind. And so I harshly begin to blame people for the circumstances that I have concluded to be the cause for my emotional upheaval. I have since learned that what I really needed was some new information. My desire to know was great indeed, but my ego never allowed me to consider that I didn't possess the knowledge that would be required for me to make some major adjustments in my attitude toward myself and mankind. When I had enough pain, and surrendered to the fact that I needed some new information, the pupil was ready and the teacher did appear.

Prayer
God, please help me remain teachable. I need to remember that knowledge alone is not power. It is in understanding where to gain the knowledge that empowers me to live and grow in my recovery. Amen

May 8

Thought for the day
Those who expect to reap the blessings of freedom must, like men, undergo the fatigue of supporting it.

Thomas Paine

Meditation
When we reach out for help for the very first time, we begin to reap the blessings of freedom from depression. As we progress in our recovery and regain control of our lives, many of us grow to expect a continuous reprieve from the symptoms of this illness. We hope that we are cured. Unfortunately, most of us who have been treating depression for any considerable length of time can attest to the fact that the probability of a sufferer never having a recurrence with the darkness is very unlikely. My experience has taught me that I need to be physically, mentally, and spiritually prepared to undergo the fatigue that is sometimes required of me to maintain my recovery and my life. It is delusional for me to consider the prospect of living with this malady yet never suffer any of the consequences that I frequently associated with it. I need to always be ready for the unexpected slip into the black hole so that I may quickly recover from the fall. Is it worth all the effort? Ask a mother who lost a child because of untreated clinical depression, a mother who lost her child by suicide.

Prayer
God, today I want to put effort into my recovery. I do not want to leave any rock unturned. Help me be rigorously honest with myself today. Remind me that my recovery will be everything I make out of it. Help me to not become complacent and cheat myself out of all that life has to offer me today. Amen

May 9

Thought for the day
It is not the years in your life but the life in your years that counts.

Adlai Stevenson

Meditation
I do not treat my depression so that I will not die. I treat it so that I may live. For years, my life was void of substance, purpose, and direction. I survived while being surrounded by thoughts of worthlessness and self-mutilation. I self-medicated myself with alcohol and cocaine, hoping that I would pass out, never to wake up again. The years in my life passed me by as I struggled with all my might to keep myself from falling to my untimely death. Many days, I barely could muster the mental defense required to wage such a battle. I often would have to beat back the idea that "if this is life, I want no part of it". Today, I can say with complete certainty that I want nothing to do with only surviving. I want to live. My depression, left untreated, will isolate me from my family and friends. It will rob me of any ability or ambition to help another human being. It will tell me that I am worthless and should do the world a favor by taking my own life. Today, I know that to be untrue. I recognize the symptoms of depression for what they are - symptoms. I believe in the support of the people in my life today, but more importantly, I believe my life is worthwhile because I can always help somebody else.

Prayer
God, today I want to live a life that is pleasing to you. While there is still time, I want to help anybody who reaches out from the black hole of despair and asks for help. I want to be less concerned with the quantity of my life, and more focused on the quality of it. Amen

May 10

Thought for the day
Life begins on the other side of despair.

Jean-Paul Sartre

Meditation
When we are depressed, it is virtually impossible to imagine
the other side. We become so blinded by our darkness, that
we can no longer envision the light of the shore. If life
begins on the other side of despair, then our lives end when
we are in despair. We become so paralyzed by our self-
hatred that we cannot participate in anything that resembles
good. Of true happiness, we can know little. To overcome
our despair seems insurmountable. If we knew how, we
would have already followed the path to enlightenment. We
are hopelessly lost in our depression...lost until we ask for
help. Today I must remember that it was not I who held the
key to the door of enlightenment. It was not I who made his
own way through the murky darkness of depression. It was
others who showed me the way. And when I slip back into
despair, it will be others who will ease my struggle and
gently set me into the light of the shore. But likewise, when
I am full of life, free from the bondage of depression, I
become the keeper of the key, the navigator to the light. We
have an awesome responsibility today. Do not take yours
lightly.

Prayer
God, I spent so many years of my life lost in the despair of
clinical depression. By your grace, I received the direction I
needed to begin my journey back to life. Help me remember
that it is by helping others that I help myself, and likewise,
others will always be there to help me. Amen

May 11

Thought for the day
The eternal quest of the individual human being is to shatter his loneliness.

Norman Cousins

Meditation
Many of us who suffer from depression know the feelings of utter loneliness. Clinical depression, with all of its accompanied mental twists, affects each of us in such a way that we can feel hopelessly alone, even in a crowded room. Left untreated, we slowly deteriorate to the point that we lose all hope of ever feeling "part of " again. We contemplate suicide as our only true escape from the desolation of our spiritless lives. Yet within each of us, there must burn an eternal desire to live, for without such a burning desire, we would have already taken our own lives. Many of us have exclaimed that we have been too afraid to commit suicide. That fear, in and of itself, is evidence of a stronger desire to live than to die. I believe that deep within the depths of our soul exists a supernatural will to survive. A will to survive on God's time, not our own. My eternal quest to shatter my loneliness began to show signs of purpose and direction once I surrendered to the fact that I did have an illness called depression and that I could not rid myself of its symptoms by my own means. Today, I can be alone, yet not feel lonely. When I need to reach out to my circle of friends, I can do so with no shame whatsoever. By treating my depression, I have improved my self-esteem to a level, which allows me to commune with my Creator. Thus, I never have to be alone again.

Prayer

God, today I pray for the lonely lost souls of the world. I pray you will inspire each and every one of them to reach out for help. I pray there will always be a helping hand ready to serve. Amen

May 12

Thought for the day
I believe that man will not merely endure: he will prevail.
He is immortal, not because he alone among creatures has an
inexhaustible voice, but because he has a soul, a spirit
capable of compassion and sacrifice and endurance.

William Faulkner

Meditation
You will not merely endure; you will prevail in your battle
with depression. You will prevail because you have a soul
that loves you, life, and God. You will prevail because you
have a spirit that loves you. You have a spirit that is capable
of all virtuous things, a spirit which not even depression can
destroy, a spirit that will live forever. Today you have the
endurance to survive a passing storm of depression because
you have faith in the rainbow that will follow. Today you
have an understanding about the symptoms of depression, an
understanding that allows you to have compassion for
yourself when you have slipped into the darkness of despair,
a compassion that allows you to quickly reach out for help.
When I am depressed, it can be awfully difficult for me to
believe that I will experience anything beyond merely
surviving another day. But the further I travel along my road
of enlightenment, the more evidence I collect to support the
idea that I am somebody today…that I deserve love, serenity,
and peace in my life, and that God does truly love and care
for me.

Prayer
God, today please allow me the courage and strength to
prevail in my battle with depression. Thank you for your
unconditional compassion and love, especially when I have
found it difficult to love myself. Today, please allow me to
know serenity and peace in my heart. Amen

May 13

Thought for the day
One of the best safeguards of our hopes, I have suggested, is to be able to mark off the areas of hopelessness and to acknowledge them, to face them directly, not with despair but with the creative intent of keeping them from polluting all the areas of possibility.

William F. Lynch

Meditation
By acceptance, we are able to mark off our areas of hopelessness and despair. When we accept our depression for what it really is, a treatable illness, we gain the power to separate our authentic self from the symptoms of the disease and safeguard our future hopes by seeking treatment. Prior to reaching out for help, my untreated depression was polluting all areas of possibility in my life. It was virtually impossible for me to maintain any sort of hope for myself when I was lost in the darkness of the black hole. I knew no way out. I was trying desperately to ignore the feelings of fear, loneliness, and despair by blaming my symptoms on my surroundings. Once I faced my shadow, not with despair but with the intent to fight the good fight and prevail, I found a renewed spirit to live and succeed. Today I have a strong faith in the process of my recovery. I am prepared for the valleys I will encounter along my journey to a happy destiny.

Prayer
God thank you for the courage I needed to face my shadow of depression. Please strengthen my resolve to prevail over this illness so that when I enter into the valleys of my journey, I may soon find myself back on the plateau of peace. Amen

May 14

Thought for the day
It wasn't raining when Noah built the ark.

Howard Ruff

Meditation
Today we must make a conscious effort to prepare ourselves for the next storm of depression that might cloud our lives. We know from our experiences that when we are consumed with the darkness of despair, it is very difficult for us to maintain the desire to take care of ourselves. The illness presents such a bleak forecast for our lives that we lose all interest in having any hope for the future. Knowing this, we must develop a recovery strategy to prepare ourselves for the next torrential downpour. It is very important that our strategy includes the support of understanding individuals, preferably people who also treat depression. I cannot emphasize enough how important my support group has been to my recovery. Other recovering people become so crucial because sometimes, when we are on a collision course with another bout with the darkness, we are incapable of seeing it coming. It can happen to us so slowly, yet before we know it, we are gone again. My circle of friends will readily point me toward a storm on the horizon and warn me to brace myself for whatever it may blow my way. Today, I enjoy doing the same for them.

Prayer
God, help me remember that my recovery requires effort and vigilance. Please shield me from becoming careless and complacent with that which I have worked so hard to obtain. Amen

May 15

Thought for the day
It is well to remember that the entire population of the universe, with one trifling exception, is composed of others.

John Andrew Holmes

Meditation
Meaning what, that I am not alone or that I'm not that important? Today I believe it is probably a little of both. It is good for me to feel important and worthy, but not to the point that I become arrogant, selfish, and conceited. It is also equally important for me to recognize that I am not alone in this world and that I am surrounded by great people who would cherish my friendship and companionship if only I would reach out to another and connect. When I am depressed, it is easy for me to feel as though I am drowning in the sea of humanity, yet nobody around me seems to be able to see me or hear my screams for help. Remembering that I am the one trifling exception in the universe does not mean that I have to become small and insignificant. It just means that I am not alone today. It means that our feelings of utter loneliness are not due to a shortage of people, but of other conditions such as being clinically depressed. Today, we all are important and need one another's support.

Prayer
God, when I am depressed, it is so easy for me to wonder why you would care about me. I consider the population of the world with all of its immediate problems and conclude that you do not have time for me. Help me never to put such limitations on you and question your love for me. Amen

146

May 16

Thought for the day
When you get to the end of your rope, tie a knot and hang on.

Unknown

Meditation
Today, no matter how bad it may get, tie a knot at the end of your rope and hang on. Don't give up right before the miracle happens. If you do, you will be denying God, yourself, and man the opportunity to create something truly wonderful in your life. If this is the worst it has ever been, count on it only getting better. If you can't think of one good reason to carry on yet another minute, think of the one life you may save by telling of how on this day, when you had given up all hope of living another day, you decided to hang on. Then tell them how you finally fought through all your shame and asked for help from people who understand and care. Tell them how you were told you did the right thing by coming out of the darkness and asking for help. Tell them how you were introduced to a whole new way of life. Tell them how you have slowly learned to like yourself again. Today, if you're at the end of your rope...tie a knot, ask for help, and then hang on.

Prayer
God thank you for seeing me through my darkest hours. Thank you for giving me the courage to finally tell somebody how truly rotten I felt and how I just wanted to die. Thank you for putting me in contact with people who understood and cared. Amen

May 17

Thought for the day
A loving person lives in a loving world. A hostile person lives in a hostile world: everyone you meet is your mirror.

Ken Keyes, Jr.

Meditation
A depressed person lives in a depressed world. A dark, suicidal, unhopeful, worthless person lives in a dark, dead, hopeless, worthless world. When we are depressed, what choices do we have? Have not all our efforts to create a world in which we can peacefully coexist failed? Have we not concluded, after all our efforts, that we were the problem and damaged beyond economical repair? Today we know that it is not the external elements of our life that make us clinically depressed. We all will experience the pains associated with living, and we will know grief, but when suicide or self-inflicted harm seem to be the only solution left, we need immediate medical attention. I meet many people who question whether they suffer from clinical depression. I certainly do not profess to be an expert on the subject, but I consider the suicide test to be an accurate barometer. If you feel like taking your own life, see a doctor immediately. If you do not have a doctor, go to the emergency room of your local hospital. You deserve to receive treatment for your illness and begin to learn how to love yourself and others, so that you can live in a loving world.

Prayer
God, I am frequently reminded that it is my attitude and outlook on life which shapes my perception of it. When I am in the darkness of despair, it is impossible for me to see the

good in the world that surrounds me. It is also very difficult to feel your presence in my life when I am lost in the black hole. Please help me remember how important it is that I treat my depression one day at a time. Amen

May 18

Thought for the day
I was taught when I was young that if people would only
love one another, all would be well with the world. This
seemed simple and very nice; but I found when I tried to put
it in practice not only that other people were seldom lovable,
but that I was not very lovable myself.

George Bernard Shaw

Meditation
I truly believe that it is impossible to love another unless you
first love yourself. Perhaps the reason why so many people
are seldom lovable is because so few have been taught to
love themselves first. I am certain that my untreated
depression had a large impact on my ability to love. I can
say with certainty that I flat-out hated myself. I felt so pitiful
and weak because I seemed to be so needy. I couldn't bear it
when my family would try to fix me because that was just
more evidence that I was broken. On occasion, I would take
a good, hard look at myself and see what I perceived as a
pitiful, worthless human being, and conclude that I needed to
take my own life. Looking back, It scares me to think how
dangerously close I was to killing myself. Today I am so
grateful I got help. What I have learned about myself and
this illness is that we are not one and the same. The
symptoms of depression are unlovable...but that does not
mean that I am not. I suffered for so long without a clue
about this illness that I have to work very hard at not falling
back into my old way of thinking. Maintaining a healthy
self-esteem tops my list of things to do today. What is
topping yours?

Prayer
God, I want nothing more than to feel love and peace in my heart. When I am depressed, I am robbed of my self-esteem. It is so difficult for me to experience joy when I am lost in the darkness of despair. Please help all of us who suffer from this malady find the daily healing that we need to experience love. Amen

May 19

Thought for the day
He who despises his own life is soon master of another's.

English proverb

Meditation
Prior to beginning treatment for my depression, I held myself
in such low regard. My inferiority complex had been a
constant companion for as long as my memory could serve
me. Consequently, as a child, I quickly learned how to act
like people whom I admired. I never wanted to be myself
because it was just too painful. At a very young age I lost
myself. I began to master the survival skill of being able to
be all things to all people. I learned and perfected so many
different personas that on occasion I would lose track of who
I was on any different day. My life became one big lie. Yet
beneath my camouflaged armor existed my conscience that
kept whispering, "they know". I feared being found out but I
didn't know what you would find if you did. As I entered
recovery, I was completely lost. I have begun the task of
unmasking. Each day that I am willing to keep an open mind
and heart, I am that much closer to no longer despising my
own life. Today we must all search fearlessly for our
authentic self. Our illness has distorted our ability to hold
ourselves in high esteem so we ran and hid behind the faces
of others. Our recovery is about no longer despising our
own life.

Prayer
God thank you for the courage and strength to throw away
the masks and begin to learn to be myself. It has not been
easy, and on some days it is very difficult not to despise my
life. Today I accept these feelings as symptoms of a
treatable illness and not the reality of who and what I am.
Amen

May 20

Thought for the day
I am as bad as the worst, but, thank God, I am as good as the best.

Walt Whitman

Meditation
When we are engulfed by our depression, we are all too familiar with feeling "as bad as the worst". It is very difficult to find one good thing to say about ourselves when we are consumed with the darkness. Despite evidence to the contrary, we will allow our minds to entertain wave after wave of self-defeating thoughts. With each passing wave, we allow ourselves to be buried by the lies of our illness. Depression denies us of the ability to see the good that exists in all of us. No matter how evil or ill equipped you may feel, you are still a creature of God, and the way I understand it, God does not make junk. I can honestly say that I have spent the majority of my life feeling as bad as the worst, with very little experience feeling as good as the best. I am certain that untreated depression had a lot to do with my inability to see any good within me. Today we must work hard at finding the good within us, and accept it as readily as we do the bad. It is very dangerous for people like us, not to work daily at improving our self-esteem and self-worth. By improving our perceptions of ourselves, we build a defense against the next wave of darkness that may overtake our lives.

Prayer
God, help me learn that I am not as rotten as I often believe I am. Show me that although I certainly do have my share of weaknesses, I also possess many positive attributes and strengths. Amen

May 21

Thought for the day
My creed is that:
Happiness is the only good.
The place to be happy is here.
The time to be happy is now.
The way to be happy is to make others so.
Robert G. Ingersoll

Meditation
Throughout the centuries, great thinkers have given us an abundant supply of contemplation on the subject of happiness. I will not attempt to add any wisdom as to how we may obtain it. What I will do is subscribe to the idea that happiness is good. And with the same conviction I will state that of true happiness we will know little if we suffer from untreated clinical depression. That being said, it becomes academic as to the action we must take if we want to experience true happiness. We must be treating our depression one day at a time. We must develop a support group that we can count on. If required, we must maintain our medications by regularly meeting with our doctor. If we are currently taking anti-depressants and desire to no longer take them, we should not attempt to do so against medical advice. But most important of all, we must make ourselves available to our fellow sufferers. Whether it is through on-line chats or in person, the greatest joy you will ever know will be the joy of helping others.

Prayer
God, help me to help others today. Amen

May 22

Thought for the day
Hatred is self-punishment.
Hosea Ballou

Meditation
My mask for depression has always been hatred displayed as rage. Whether I want to destroy myself or somebody else, the underlying feelings are always those of self-contempt. I have been consumed with hatred most of my life. I have been burdened by bitterness and resentment toward my family, blaming them constantly for my ill feelings. If only they would behave as I wished, then I would not feel so depressed. At times I felt so evil and ungodly that I knew if I died at that moment, I would descend straight to hell and burn for eternity. After a period of time, my mask of rage would fall. What would be revealed was a fearful, depressed man who now only hated himself and wished to die. My recovery has taught me the futility of the mask of rage. When I am really scared, I still put on the mask, but it does not take long for me to realize that I am causing myself unnecessary pain. I know it is a lie and will only cause more problems. Today I must work very hard to remain free from resentment. Accepting my depression as an illness and not the result of somebody else's behavior is a big step toward freedom from anger and self-punishment.

Prayer
God, please teach me how to remain free from anger and self-punishment today. Allow me to understand the virtues of patience, tolerance, and forgiveness. Amen

May 23

Thought for the day
A man can stand a lot as long as he can stand himself. He can live without hope, without friends, without books, even without music, as long as he can listen to his own thoughts.

Axel Munthe

Meditation
What will your thoughts consist of today? Will they be reassuring and nurturing or will they be self-destructive? For the longest time I did not have much of a choice as to the type of thoughts I would entertain. I would try to look on the brighter side of things, wanting desperately to believe that life wasn't that bad. Unfortunately, I often would fail terribly at my attempts to have a more positive outlook on life. I would become so angry with myself because I felt like I should have been able to change my thoughts to better reflect the reality that was my life. It was absolutely maddening to be consumed with thoughts of self-destruction, self-pity, and suicide when there was nothing happening in my life that would support my claims to agony. I could not stand to be in my own mind any more. I could not rely on my own thinking because it was, I concluded, completely insane. Today, although it is not easy, I am able to stop my abusive thinking when I start telling someone in my circle of support exactly how I am thinking. I have to be completely honest with them, telling them all of the insanity that is running rampant in my head. By doing so, they are able to supply me with some desperately needed positive affirmation and usually a little comic relief. They help to take the power and control away from the illness and put it back in my hands. They tell me that I no longer have to abuse myself with self-defeating thoughts.

Prayer
God, help me continue to learn how to rid my mind quickly of self-defeating thoughts. Teach me to remain rigorously honest with my friends in recovery so they may continue to channel your love and grace to me. Amen

May 24

Thought for the day
I never found the companion that was so companionable as
solitude.

Henry David Thoreau

Meditation
What an absolute joy it has been for me to experience
solitude instead of loneliness. I never understood the
difference until I reached a point in my recovery when I
looked forward to the time that I could be completely alone
with my thoughts for no other purpose then to pray for
guidance and inspiration and to listen to my inner voice. We
are all too familiar with the need to isolate ourselves from
the rest of the world when we are depressed. To be isolated
when depressed is probably one of the coldest, emptiest,
loneliest feelings I have ever experienced. Also, it was
probably one of the most dangerous moments in my life.
Most people who take their own lives do so when they are
alone. Today when I am depressed, it is of the utmost
importance that I surround myself with understanding
people, but once my mood is stabilized, it is equally
important that I enjoy the rewards of recovery by allowing
myself time for silent solitude.

Prayer
God, it can be very difficult for me to make the time that I
need to enjoy solitude in my life. Help me keep my
priorities in perspective so I may make the time I need to
continue my spiritual journey. Amen

May 25

Thought for the day
You are loved. If so, what else matters?

Edna St. Vincent Millay

Meditation
You are loved. Whether you feel it or believe you are worthy of it, somebody loves and cares deeply about you. You may not even know the person, yet there are many wonderful people in this world who are already praying for your well-being and happiness. You probably will not have to search the world over to find such a person. They may be members of your immediate family or a close friend. Perhaps a concerned neighbor or a member of your local church is praying for your recovery. Don't be mistaken by the negative self-talk that depression brings about in your mind. When I am at my lowest, darkest moments, I often look at a little note that was handed to me years ago by a total stranger, at the beginning of my recovery journey. All it says is, "Remember, somebody is praying for you." Today, what else matters?

Prayer
God, help me remember that I am loved by so many people. When I am in my valley of darkness, remind me that, although I may not feel it or believe it, I am loved. Amen

May 26

Thought for the day
God hasn't called me to be successful. He's called me to be faithful.

Mother Teresa

Meditation
As a person who suffers from clinical depression, I have observed that when I experience what "normal" people would consider a sad or depressing event, I often become paralyzed with self-pity and self-contempt. My threshold for such events seems to be lower than that of non-sufferers, consequently it appears as if I am overreacting and being melodramatic when I happen to be caught in one of life's more painful moments. As a knee-jerk reaction to defend myself against such unpleasant experiences, I set about trying to control all things that could affect my life. One of my greatest pursuits to defend myself against unpleasant experiences was to be materially successful. I thought that if I had a lot of money, I would be happy and happy people have far fewer problems than unhappy people do, right? My experiences in life have now taught me otherwise. Today I know that my success has nothing to do with money. It has to do only with being faithful to myself and my God. I have also accepted that success is not a destination, it is a work in progress. I remain faithful to myself when I remain faithful to the work.

Prayer
God, my recovery has opened my eyes to so many new ideas, new ways for me to define myself and the world in which I live. I pray that I will continue to take advantage of every opportunity you provide me so I may continue to grow spiritually and mentally. Amen

May 27

Thought for the day
May you live all the days of your life.

Jonathan Swift

Meditation
When we are consumed with the persistent pessimism
known as clinical depression, we are not living life at all.
We are merely surviving yet another day in our own mental
hell. Millions of us have lived in the darkness for so long
that we recoil from the light. We are scared to death of the
idea of feeling good again. The letdowns are more than we
can bear, so we stay stuck in the darkness of despair and self-
destruction. There is an element of safety in familiarity,
whether it is harmful or not. As our condition goes
undiagnosed for perhaps years, we suffer grave losses. Lost
opportunities to spend with our family, lost opportunities at a
career we may have dreamed of pursuing, lost spouses
through separation and divorce because neither party really
understood what the cause of the disenchantment was with
each other. Haven't we suffered enough? You do deserve
the best that life has to offer. If you do not believe this
today, get some help. Life is too short. Before you know it,
it will pass you by. It is time that we live all the remaining
days of our lives. Our depression has taken enough.

Prayer
God, I want to live the rest of my life to its fullest. I want to
seize each day with excitement, enchantment, and hope.
Amen

May 28

Thought for the day
Anger helps straighten out a problem like a fan helps straighten out a pile of papers.

Susan Marcotte

Meditation
I have learned, in my recovery, that I do not have the luxury of "justifiable anger". Oh, I still like to intimidate and manipulate others by allowing them to see that I am extremely agitated with their behavior and that I am about to lose all control and spin into a despicable rage if they do not quickly mend their ways. The problem with that behavior today is that I know it is totally unacceptable and solves nothing. I am also acutely aware that my anger is usually a "cover up" for sadness or depression. As I have progressed along my path, I have learned to sort through my rage and quickly get to the root of the problem. Sometimes I am experiencing many different emotions as a result of some "trigger" being set off within me. Other times I find that I am only covering up symptoms of depression. By working through our thoughts and emotions, we are able to constructively pursue resolution to our problems and ill feelings without the rubble to sweep up after a fit of rage. There was a time in my life when, if it were breakable, I would break it. I am so grateful I no longer have to live like that.

Prayer
God, help me continue to learn how to quickly sort through all my feelings. Show me how to get at the root of what is disturbing me so I may find relief in an appropriate way. Amen

162

May 29

Thought for the day
Inches make champions.

Vince Lombardi

Meditation
My recovery from depression has been a slow, tedious process. Just when I think I got it beat...I've lapsed back into an unexplainable period of feeling doomed. These episodes initially seem like failure to me. That of course, only adds to my depressed outlook on life. But each time I recover from the darkness, I enjoy a renewed sense of hope. I have to remember not to allow myself to believe that I am going to remain free from depression for the rest of my life. I have suffered many setbacks during my recovery. I have had to switch medications repeatedly. I have worked very hard at cleaning up the wreckage of my past in the hope of making my life more livable today. I believe that all of my efforts were not in vain. Although living with depression is sometimes very painful, it is still better than dying from it. It is important that I reward myself for the progress that I have made. By all accounts I should be dead. I need to remain diligent and faithful to the process, and be happy with the progress that I make, even if it is only one inch at a time.

Prayer
God, help me become patient with my progress. Allow me the wisdom to accept the fact that I will probably have to deal with depressed setbacks the rest of my life. Grant me the courage to purposefully continue on. Amen

May 30

Thought for the day
Begin at the beginning, go on till you come to the end, and
then stop.

Lewis Carroll

Meditation
There are days when my problems seem insurmountable.
The bed is unmade, there are dishes in the sink, my car won't
start, the checking account is empty, and my life is a
worthless waste. Deep in my heart, if I listen, I can hear the
voice telling me that this is my disease talking to me, filling
my head with lies, robbing me of this most precious day. I
try to focus on one thing. Doing those dishes, or making the
bed. If I can do just one positive thing in the face of my
depression, the next becomes a little easier. Before I know
it, I have come to the end of my tasks and the end of my day.
My heart is a little lighter. I know once again that God is
looking out for me.

Prayer
God, help me to do just one good thing today, and take pride
in it. Help me remember that I will have days when getting
up out of bed is a major accomplishment. If I can then turn
around and make that bed, I have pushed my disease of
depression back another notch. Amen

May 31

Thought for the day
He has served who now and then
Has helped along his fellowman.
Edgar A. Guest

Meditation
Today I cannot afford to allow my recovery to become a spectator sport. I must be active in my pursuit to help others who may be in dire need of a lending hand or a gentle ear. My spiritual condition is improved by serving others, much more so than by being served by others. When I am depressed, it is very important for me to "get out of myself" and be with understanding people who will help me take care of myself. Likewise, I need to be willing and able to support someone else during his or her time of struggle. I know this to be God's will for me today.

Prayer
God, help me lose interest in selfish things so that I may gain interest in helping others. Amen

June 1

Thought for the day
Resolve to be thyself; and know that who finds himself, loses his misery.

Matthew Arnold

Meditation
By the grace of God, I have slowly learned who I am and, as importantly, who I am not. I have experienced little moments of self-discovery...moments that have overwhelmed me with the joy and certainty that I finally have my life on the right track. As my self-awareness begins to grow, I have noticed that my overall miserable outlook has lessened. Today I realize that I must continue to search through my thoughts and actions...to measure my motives, to purge my heart of impurities, and to weed my mind of harmful thinking.

Prayer
God, for years I lived without any true knowledge of what was actually wrong with me. I struggled so hard to live and feel right, but I always was left with feelings of worthlessness and despair. Today, by your grace, I have a solid foundation from which I can now build my character upon. Amen

June 2

Thought for the day
The purpose of learning is growth, and our minds, unlike our bodies, can continue growing as we continue to live.

Mortimer Adler

Meditation
Having spent the better part of the last sixteen years of my life struggling to develop some semblance of normalcy, I have acquired a slew of professional opinions as to what it is that ails me. At times, because of my eager pursuit to rid myself of all that seemed wrong, I ended up with "information overload" and would not have a clear direction as to what the next right move should be. It is very easy for me to become overwhelmed with what appears to be a monstrous maze that I must negotiate if I ever hope to achieve serenity and peace in my life. Today it is important that I find focus and balance in my pursuit of new information. Growth is essential to my life, but just like a beautiful garden, too much water can drown it. I need a well of information to draw upon, but I need not use it all at once. And likening my recovery to a garden, I need to focus my efforts toward maintaining all that is well and applying a little extra effort wherever there may appear to be wilting. I believe that learning may lead to growth, but today the biggest challenge for me is to be able to weed and separate the valuable information from all that is a liability to me.

Prayer
God, help me today to have the wisdom not to subscribe to erroneous information. Help me continue toward personal growth and nurture the garden of my mind by maintaining all that is well while weeding out all that is harmful. Amen

June 3

Thought for the day
People are always blaming their circumstances for being
what they are. The people who get on in this world are the
people who get up and look for the circumstances they want,
and if they can't find them, make them.

George Bernard Shaw

Meditation
The most meaningful circumstances that occur in my life
today are those that I create from within. My recovery has
taught me that not only can I change the circumstances
within me, but that I must. We are all too familiar with the
blaming game. We have played it for so long that whenever
we start to feel depressed and discontent, we immediately
start to search for somebody or something to blame for our
condition. Today, if I want to get along in this world, I must
get up and create some new circumstances within myself. I
must change all of my negative self-talk, which upon closer
examination always turns out to be half-truths or complete
lies, and replace these self-defeating messages with honest
thinking. I also must be prepared for the inevitable times
when I am depressed and unable to create the circumstances
that I desire. At these moments, in order to make the
circumstances that are needed for my well-being, I have to
ask for help.

Prayer
God, today I must remember that I may not be able to change
all of the circumstances that surround me, but I can change
my inner circumstances at anytime. By doing so, I will find
that the events outside of me lose their power to push me
around. Please give me the courage and strength to continue
to improve upon my inner self. Amen

June 4

Thought for the day
We judge ourselves by what we feel we are capable of doing, while others judge us by what we have already done.
Henry Wadsworth Longfellow

Meditation
Until I was able to understand this, I spent a great deal of my life feeling very "bad". Growing up in a dysfunctional household without the benefit of a simple education on life, I was always struggling with feelings of inadequacy because of people maintaining their judgements of my mistakes, instead of helping me move toward my new ideas. As a result, I often would think that there was something wrong with me, so I would revert back to dwelling on my old mistakes and then begin the endearing act of beating myself up without mercy. Is it any wonder I felt bad? I now know, through treatment and the help of others that my mistakes are just that...mistakes. If I can begin to focus on my future and implement what I have learned from my trials and tribulations, I can change what I feel I am capable of doing into something I've already done. By doing so, I increase my self-worth, and the other people in my life will begin to focus more on my accomplishments rather than my errors. This does require a critical component to be successful...the support of reliable, understanding people. If you do not have the support of your family, then you must reach out to somebody else. If you know you need someone, give yourself this gift today. If your disease tells you that there is no one there for you, realize that this message is simply your depression attempting to keep you isolated yet another day.

Prayer
God, please grant me the wisdom to discern between the disease of depression and the reality of your gifts that are available to me. Let me accept your gifts today without further hesitation and use them in a way that is pleasing to you. Amen

June 5

Thought for the day
I am not responsible for my feelings – only for what I do with them.

Dr. Ceophus Martin

Meditation
Today, if you ask me how I am feeling, I will probably rattle off to you a list of emotions. For example, I know that when I feel angry there is also some other emotions lurking beneath my seething disposition. Usually, if I am taking care of myself by self-examination, I will discover fear as the root of my indignant air. It is my responsibility to then rid myself of the superficial anger and turn my attention to my fearfulness. By getting honest with myself and getting to the root of a feeling, I can much more accurately make the adjustments in my attitude that are necessary to improve my emotional and spiritual condition. I remember how awestruck I was when I was first told that I could dismiss my negative thinking and feelings and replace them with a positive outlook. What I was not told was how difficult it could be sometimes to do this. Today, I must be willing to make a conscious effort to accurately identify how I feel, and then replace any negative, painful thoughts with positive ones.

Prayer
God, throughout my day I will be bombarded with feelings that are not factual. Please give me the insight to accurately appraise how I am feeling, and then the courage to adjust my attitude accordingly. Amen

June 6

Thought for the day
And behold you were within me, and I out of myself, and there I searched for you.

St. Augustine

Meditation
The spiritual bankruptcy that we experience when we are suffering from depression is devastating. If we normally possess a faith in a loving, forgiving God, that belief frequently becomes foreign and unidentifiable in the darkness of the black hole. The illness devours all our hopes and tells us that nobody, including God, cares about us. We feel as though we cannot turn to God in our present condition because we believe that we are unworthy of his saving grace. We feel as though we have to elevate ourselves out of the darkness before God will hear from us. And so we search aimlessly for relief from our pain, grabbing at anything that has the resemblance of "normal". But today we may see and believe that our Creator is within us at all times. We can accept and understand that our feelings of worthlessness are a symptom of an illness and not a true appraisal of our value to mankind. We can ask God for help at anytime, especially in the darkness of the black hole.

Prayer
God, it is easy for me to become lost in my pursuit of serenity and peace. I can become distracted by so many worldly things, that I begin to look for you in all the wrong places. Please continue to shepherd me so I may not stray far from your flock. Amen

June 7

Thought for the day
Genuine self love is the greatest protection against dependent relationships.

Robert Coleman

Meditation
We have learned that when we are depressed, we lack self-love. As a result of this deficiency in our character, we become extremely needy people. Because we are unable to validate ourselves, it becomes necessary for us to find approval from other people. The problem arises when we do not receive from others what we lack in ourselves. The expectation is flawed to begin with because the problem lies within. Yet, as a result of our ignorance in regard to the illness of clinical depression, we spend years forging abusive, dependent relationships. Never achieving the feelings of fulfillment, we become abusive to the very people we expect to make us feel loved. And so the spiral downward continues, destroying relationships, and leaving all involved feeling angry, betrayed, and victimized. Today I must continue to nurture myself by practicing self-love. By doing so, I can protect myself from dependent relationships and develop healthy behaviors.

Prayer
God, please help me remain free from abusive, dependent relationships. Help me continue to learn how to love myself so I may avoid placing unrealistic expectations on the people I love. Amen

June 8

Thought for the day
As long as habit and routine dictate the pattern of living, new dimensions of the soul will not emerge.

Henry Van Dyke

Meditation
Changing a deeply entrenched pattern of behavior...a behavior that we have repeated over and over throughout the course of our lives, is not an easy task. Having been depressed for so long, nurturing all those menacing, self-defeating thoughts, we find it difficult to foster a positive outlook on life. Our chances of success in recovery are directly proportional to our desire and ability to learn and practice new ways of thinking and living. I certainly will not argue with the fact that I desperately was in need of a new dimension of existence. My soul could not emerge from under the weight of my despair until I considered and accepted that my behaviors were the symptoms of an illness. In so doing, I was able to lighten my burden enough to begin to exercise some new and exciting options as to how I could live my life.

Prayer
God thank you for showing me how to break my destructive patterns of behavior. Help me continue to guard myself against slipping into my old mind traps. If I do happen to lapse into old behavior, please help me recognize it immediately and then use the skills I have learned to get back on the right track. Amen

June 9

Thought for the day
Lives of great men all remind us
We can make our lives sublime
And, departing, leave behind us
footprints on the sands of time.
Henry Wadsworth Longfellow

Meditation
When we are filled with feelings of worthlessness, we cannot believe we could be anything other than a failure. Convincing ourselves that we can't, shouldn't, or don't deserve it, even if there is no evidence to support our defective claim, we reluctantly proceed with our lives, certain to leave nothing but pain in our wake. Upon accepting and treating our depression as an illness, not as a flawed character, we begin to realize that we are not as "broken" as we once thought. We find that we can make a difference in the lives of people we come in contact with. We probably will not achieve stardom, although some of us might, but we do learn that even the smallest act of generosity or kindness can make a large footprint on the beaches of life.

Prayer
God, when I am suffering from depression, I lose all faith that I have any true value. Help me remember that by my experiences with this illness, I am in a position to help others who also suffer, and this is truly a blessing. Amen

June 10

Thought for the day
Loneliness expresses the pain of being alone and solitude expresses the glory of being alone.

Paul Tillich

Meditation
The glory of being alone. My recovery from depression has allowed me to experience solitude for perhaps the first time in my life. I recall as a child, feeling extremely afraid of being left by myself. I felt very uncertain and unsafe when alone. As I grew older, I expected that I would outgrow my childish fears. But I did not. It seemed that the older I got, the more frightened I became when left to my own devices. The insanity of all of this was that my untreated depression isolated me from other people, and left me feeling alone, even in their presence. Thus, I became a hyper-vigilant, paranoid person who masked his fears with anger and rage followed by deep, dark trips to the black hole. Thanks to God and a whole lot of support from some wonderful people, I no longer have to live life looking through my rear-view mirror. As a result of my recovery, I can look forward to the times that I can be alone. I have learned that I can be great company during my moments of solitude.

Prayer
God, my recovery has given me a new lease on life. Today I no longer have to live with the fear of being alone. I have a wonderful circle of friends who understand depression as an illness, who are always there for me. By consistently striving to improve my faith in you, the recovery process, my friends, and myself, I am now able to enjoy the glory of solitude. Amen

June 11

Thought for the day
God offers to every mind its choice between truth and repose. Take which you please-you can never have both.
Ralph Waldo Emerson

Meditation
Denial is a contemptuous corrosive that erodes the clarity of truth. God may in fact offer every mind its choice between truth and lies, but for me, the distinction between the two has not always been so readily definable. How many times have we acted on what we believed to be the truth, only to find out later that it was a lie? Often I have felt as if what I really had to choose between was lies or half-truths. When I am suffering from clinical depression, I am living a lie. Before I was diagnosed with this illness, I did not know that my reactions to the symptoms of this illness were not based on the truth. I felt absolutely justified in my negative, abusive thinking. I convinced myself that the grievances that I had, and proclaimed as the cause of my words and actions, were completely accurate. I never considered that maybe I was wrong. Today I realize that God offers to every *healthy* mind these two choices. When I am in the grips of depression, it is best that I not become too headstrong as to why I feel depressed, because nine chances out of ten, I will be wrong. Usually it is because I am exhibiting the symptoms of an illness, and nothing else.

Prayer
God thank you for the wisdom that helps me have the insight to clearly identify the truths in my life. Remind me when I am depressed, that life is not what it may appear to be, and that I am best to wait until my depression ends before I draw any conclusions about myself or the world in which I live. Amen

June 12

Thought for the day
We may be the only Easter lily some people ever see.

Rev. R. Oelerich

Meditation
Believe it or not, it may be true. We come into contact with
people throughout our day...mostly with total strangers.
When we are depressed, we might find ourselves grudgingly
walking through our local supermarket to pick up the
necessity that dragged us out of our self-imposed isolation.
With our heads hung low, we desperately avoid eye contact
with any passerby. As we stand in the hellishly slow
checkout line, we begin to observe the ease and joy others
seem to be experiencing. We compulsively react by
grabbing a family size bag of self-pity and a case of self-
contempt and throw it into our cart. The check out person is
grotesquely overflowing with enthusiasm and happiness. I
usually feel sorry for such a person who obviously does not
have the first clue about how absolutely wretched life really
is. As I depart the store with my dark cloud of despair
looming close above, I see an old friend heading in my
direction. Anxiety rushes through me as I use a passing car
to run interference so that I may make it to my car
undetected. I rush home to the safety of my hell. As I look
back on the many similar experiences that I had encountered,
I can't help but notice that God had placed along my path
many Easter lilies that I chose to ignore. Today I have a
strong faith in the spiritual implications of chance
encounters. I need to hold my head up and look the world in
the eye. By doing so I may enjoy the lilies and become one
myself.

Prayer

God, when I am depressed, I miss out on so many joys. With my head held low, I cannot experience all the wonderful simplicities of life that you have placed before me. Today, no matter how badly I may feel, help me keep my head up so I do not miss seeing the Easter lilies. Amen

June 13

Thought for the day
Who's afraid of the big bad wolf?
Walt Disney

Meditation
Depression is like a wolf sometimes. It stalks us relentlessly. It cuts us off from our friends and family and tries to isolate us in the darkness. And, finally, it tries to take our life. The way I keep the "wolf" from my door is by remembering that I have a disease called depression that needs to be treated daily. I take my medication when required. I stay with my "herd" of family and friends, keeping in close contact with them. I work my program, if I have a history of addiction and self-medication. Most of all, I try not to stray from my Shepherd, for he, more than anything else will keep me safe.

Prayer
God, you are my shepherd. Lead me to the green meadows and still waters of health. With you I know I need fear nothing. Amen

June 14

Thought for the day
The price of wisdom is above rubies.
Job 28:18

Meditation
The price of wisdom is the price of my life. For years I
worked extremely hard at amassing wealth. Certain that I
would be happy through acquisition, I plotted, schemed, and
manipulated myself into positions of authority and notoriety.
Peculiarly, at my highest moments of monetary success, I
felt the most uncertain about myself. As my bouts with
depression intensified, my resolve to succeed in life
dwindled. I soon reached a point in my life where I was
convinced that I was doomed to failure. During my lowest,
darkest moments, defining success as a monetary conquest
rather than a spiritual peace, I attempted to take my own life.
By the grace of God I lived to tell the tale of how misguided
my perception of life truly was. Today I realize that
although financial security does have its merit, it does not
determine my worth as a human being...that the most valued
entity in my life today is wisdom. The wisdom and insight
that I have gained through my recovery process has saved
my life. That wisdom is truly above all the rubies in the
world.

Prayer
God, I lived my life for so long with a distorted perception of
how I could achieve happiness. Through recovery I have
learned that the inner peace I sought to purchase was never
for sale. Today help me remember that the true joy of life
lies within my heart. Amen

June 15

Thought for the day
Only with a true friend's input can we hope to see our world
clearly, for our own perception always seems the truth.

Dr. Richard Fritz

Meditation
The illness of clinical depression is a disease of distorted
perceptions. When we are depressed, wallowing in our own
self-perceived worthlessness, the truth about the environment
in which we live is hidden behind the dark clouds of despair.
I cannot count the times in my life when my perceptions of
reality were thrown off course by an unexpected trip into the
black hole. Worst of all, when I am lost in the darkness, I
am usually the last person to realize it. Everyone that I come
in contact with can tell that something is weighing very
heavily on my mind. If they ask, I will readily tell them all
the reasons that I feel so rotten. Usually my punishment
does not fit the crime. People will say things like, "lighten
up" or "you're overreacting again". Of course these type of
comments only fan the flames of self-contempt. These good
people do not mean us any harm. They are trying to help,
they just don't know how. That is why it is so important to
my recovery that I have true friends in my life...friends who
understand the struggles that are associated with depression.
When I am depressed, it will usually be one of my friends
who will notice the symptoms and tell me, "You're
depressed". By doing so, they help me to extinguish the fire
of self-contempt and begin to treat my illness correctly.

Prayer
God thank you for the true friends I have in my life today.
There have been many times over the past years, when my
friends were there to see me through the darkness of

depression.   Help me remember that it is also my responsibility to always be there for them if they begin to exhibit the symptoms of this illness. Amen

June 16

Thought for the day
The lust for power, for dominating others, inflames the heart
more than any other passion.

Tacitus

Meditation
As a person who unknowingly suffered from clinical
depression for years, I became a very dominating,
controlling person...not out of passion but out of fear. My
fears of abandonment and failure were so intense that, out of
sheer desperation, I had to be in control of all relationships
and outcomes of events. If I could not be certain that events
would unfold as I required, I would totally avoid them. The
lust for power, for dominating others is as deceptive as
depression itself. Today, if I am not taking care of myself, I
can still lapse into a "power trip" and attempt to control
another person's thoughts and behavior. The outcome
always will leave me feeling bewildered and angry. Today I
have found that my life is most enjoyable when I stay in the
moment and focus on my own behaviors, leaving everyone
else's lives in the more capable hands of God.

Prayer
God, please help me focus on my own recovery. Help me
remember that my "power trips" have always taken me to a
dead end. Amen

June 17

Thought for the day
Man's loneliness is but his fear of life.

Eugene O'Neill

Meditation
As I spiraled downward into that deep dark abyss of depression, I could only imagine what could be awaiting me at the bottom of the pit. My dreams became nightmares and my nightmares became realities. Sometimes I didn't know if night was day or day was night. I felt like I was sinking in a pool of quicksand, left alone to die. Fear and self-loathing were my only companions. Suicidal thoughts raced through my head. I wished for the end, but was too scared to take my own life. In a brief moment of clarity after I cried out to God for help, I was able to rise and call a counselor that I had previously worked with. He referred me to a treatment facility because of my suicidal thoughts. I was put on medication, and for the first time, I was able to get honest about some issues that had been haunting me for years. Today, if the need arises, I will return to therapy for a period of time, leaving my ego and false pride at the door. I must remain ever vigilant in my fight against depression because it would rather see me dead. Today, I don't have to drag myself through life dreading waking up each day. I can truly be happy, joyous, and free.

Prayer
God, please grant me the strength to cope with whatever obstacles stand in my path today. Please give me the strength to take whatever steps are necessary to treat my depression. Amen

June 18

Thought for the day
The good life is a process, not a state of being.   It is a
direction, not a destination.

Carl Rogers

Meditation
I have worked very hard to relieve myself of the "all or
nothing" thinking that has plagued my life.   I was always
trying to arrive, yet I never got there.   To me it seemed as
though God kept moving the finish line.   Recovery from
depression is definitely an ongoing daily process.   Once I
accepted my reality, treating this illness became much
simpler.   I no longer have to feel like a failure when I
experience another period of darkness in my life.   I have
been given the tools to succeed; now it is up to me to use
them to the best of my ability.

Prayer
God, help me be patient with my progress as I trudge along
this road called life.   Please show me your direction, and
allow me serenity and peace as I make my way through the
process. Amen

June 19

Thought for the day
I have sometimes been wildly, despairingly, acutely miserable, but through it all I still know quite certainly that just being <u>alive</u> is a grand thing.

Agatha Christie

Meditation
There were times when I was imprisoned so tightly in my own endless night that being alive was far from a grand thing...it was an almost unbearable burden. I was certain that the world would be a much better place without me, and that I would be much better off without the world. But somewhere, somehow, my Higher Power spoke to me and gave me the strength to make a small step forward – to pick up the telephone, to confide in a friend, to make that appointment. That first small step was followed by other steps, and eventually I realized that to be alive was a grand thing. My life has hope and purpose now. And when I feel the cold fog of depression rolling back in, I know that God is there for me and that he will show me the way out - again.

Prayer
God, when I am overwhelmed by the weight of life...help me remember its beauty and lightness. Help me move back into the light. Amen

June 20

Thought for the day
Of course I prayed-and did God care?
He cared as much as on the air
A bird had stamped her foot
And cried, "Give me!"
Emily Dickinson

Meditation
I recall that in my darkest hour I began to journal my prayers, believing that if I wrote them down on paper they would have a better chance of being heard by the Almighty. Prior to writing my prayers, I was certain that my bedroom ceiling was a prayer deflector, so I would walk outside and speak to the sky. I often felt as though all my praying was for naught. It has been said that more things are wrought through prayer than most people realize, yet I wasn't seeing God working in my life at all. That is not to say that God wasn't listening to me anymore, it is to say that I was too sick to see or comprehend what God had in store for me. When I look back on the events in my life that finally landed me in the hospital, I can say with complete certainty that I could not have ever dreamt up the scenario that played out. If I would have received what I was praying for, when I was praying for it, I might very well be dead today. God does work in ways that I may never understand, but today, it is still best for me to allow God to be God and me to be me.

Prayer
God thank you for your everlasting love and compassion. Thank you for working in my life, even when I have lost all faith in you. Amen

June 21

Thought for the day
It is easy to bring others down to your level instead of
bringing yourself up to their level, but it is never ever right.
Chen Fawn Meng

Meditation
I can look back on my life prior to recovery and realize that
the times that I was having fun or laughing, it was usually at
someone else's expense. My self -esteem had sunk so low,
that I had to pick on others to make me feel good about
myself. I had become a black belt at verbal karate. I could
cut people to ribbons with my mouth. I had also become an
expert at body language and facial expressions to drive
people away from me. I didn't want anyone to get close to
me, because after all, if you got to know me, you wouldn't
like me. This was the kind of lie that I told myself. As I
progressed in my recovery, I found that the more I was able
to take interest in the problems of others, the smaller my
problems became. In helping others I had begun to help
myself. I had become so self-centered that I thought the
whole world revolved around me. I have since found that it
wasn't all about me and that my greatest rewards were
received by being of maximum service to God and others
without seeking anything in return. This is one of the great
spiritual axioms.

Prayer
God, please remove from me the selfishness and self-
centeredness that stand in the way of my being of service to
you and others. Please mold me into the spiritual being that I
was meant to be. Amen

June 22

Thought for the day
Often the test of courage is not to die, but to live.

Orestes

Meditation
How courageous we truly are...we who suffer from clinical depression. To do battle with the depressed thoughts of this illness requires incredible stamina and intestinal fortitude. To not fold under the immense strain of feeling worthless and suicidal is evidence of our true boldness and guts. Millions upon millions of us have taken a stand against this agonizing disease and said, " No longer!" No longer will I allow myself to be engulfed with self-pity and abusive thinking. No longer will I allow my mind to be host to the worm of mental and spiritual death. It would have been cowardly and selfish to take the easy way out by committing suicide. We chose to test our courage by fighting on. Today we should hold our heads high and be proud of who we are and reward ourselves for how far we have come. If you are currently fighting a bout with depression, fight on. If you currently have your depression in check, help somebody who is suffering to fight on. If you are just beginning your journey and are scared, call out for reinforcements. We will be there to help you fight on. Thank God, today we all have the courage to live.

Prayer
God thank you for the courage to live. Today there are millions of people who are still suffering from this illness because they do not understand it, or they are too afraid to admit it. Grant them the courage to take that huge first step by asking for help. Amen

190

June 23

Thought for the day
Great men are they who see the spiritual is stronger than any
material force, that thoughts rule the world.

Ralph Waldo Emerson

Meditation
I imagine that if all the thoughts of all who suffer from
clinical depression were harnessed and released upon the
world simultaneously, the earth would shatter into billions of
tiny pieces that would then throw themselves into the fiery
sun. Our thoughts when depressed are thoughts of hate and
self-destruction. Of spiritual things, we can know very little.
We become so absorbed with self-pity that the idea of a
loving God who cares about our well being is ludicrous. As
we enter recovery, we begin to emerge from the darkness of
despair for perhaps the first time in years. We begin to learn
new techniques to cope with our illness. We begin to believe
in our heart that the spiritual is much stronger and more
relevant to our lives than any material force. As we
progress, we soon realize that our thoughts were killing us.
A large part of my recovery today is to continuously
challenge my thoughts, attitudes, and ideas to ensure that I
am living within the framework of reality and not within the
darkness of depression. By soliciting the help of my friends,
I can more readily make the spiritual connection and discard
the forces of the material world.

Prayer
God, help me not to be deceived by the forces of the material
world. Help me keep the true value of material things in its
proper perspective. Show me the way to live a spiritual life.
Amen

June 24

Thought for the day
Love cures people. Both the ones who give it, and the ones who receive it.

Karl Menninger

Meditation
The healing power of feeling loved is indescribable and measureless. For many of us who have suffered for so long from untreated clinical depression, the feeling of being loved can bring us to shed tears of joy upon first contact with its overwhelming power. When we are in the black hole, we are not in a position to receive love and we certainly are in no position to give any either. If our condition persists, we become desperate to feel better. We begin to look for relief outside of ourselves. Being deprived of feeling affection for so long, we become angry with our family when they fail to make us feel their warmth and admiration. Of course today we know that even if our family did their best to convince us that we were lovable, we would not have accepted it because we were convinced otherwise. As our depression subsides, we begin to develop a renewed spirit toward love. We learn that love does cure people. We understand today that we are better off to begin loving others and ourselves than to wait for somebody to love us.

Prayer
God, in my recovery process I have been told that I would be loved until I could love myself. Although I am certain love was present in my life, I was never able to feel it until I was able to love myself. Today, help me love somebody until they are stable enough to love them self. Amen

June 25

Thought for the day
Worry never robs tomorrow of its sorrow; it only saps today
of its strength.   **A.J. Cronin**

Meditation
We gain no advantage over future events by worrying about
them. They are coming whether we like it or not. We are all
guilty of worrying about things that are out of our control.
When we are suffering from depression, our lives are
overshadowed by our perceived sense of impending doom.
We take our worries about such things and convince
ourselves that they are already our reality. We develop
presumptuous resentments toward people, places, and
things...certain that the pain we imagine they will cause us
will come to pass. We use our worries to bolster our claim
that we are justified for acting and feeling the way we do.
The reality is our worries never catch up with us because we
are always worrying about the tomorrow that never comes.
Today is the tomorrow you were worried about yesterday.
Are you worried about today, or have you already started
worrying about tomorrow, next week, next month, or next
year? And if you are living in the future, who is looking out
for you today? Recovery is a process. To rid ourselves of
destructive, wasteful, fruitless behavior takes practice. Many
people have found that living one day at a time is more than
a catchy slogan, it is a great way of life. Today, try to set
your worries aside and just focus on living in this day. You
may be surprised at what pleasures you can find living in the
now.

Prayer
God, today please help me live in the now. Help me avoid
wasting my energy worrying about things that are out of my
control. Amen

June 26

Thought for the day
The endeavor, in all branches of knowledge, is to see the object as in itself it really is.

Matthew Arnold

Meditation
When I finally was brought to my knees by untreated clinical depression, I quickly learned that what I thought I knew and understood about myself was erroneous information. God put a great man in my life who was quick to point out to me that what I was in desperate need of was some new information. When I became willing to listen and learn, I quickly realized that what I thought was my problem was not my problem at all. Out of complete ignorance about the disease of depression, I developed a lengthy list of lies and perceptions that I held as truths. It is a painful experience to acknowledge that lifelong ideas and concepts, creeds by which I had lived my life, were not only causing me harm by keeping me in a delusional state of mind, they were constant falsehoods by which I was living my life. Today, through introspection and a learned intuitiveness, I am constantly gaining new knowledge...knowledge that has helped me to discover who I truly am.

Prayer
God, I lived so many lies for so many years that I must work very hard at uncovering the truths about who I am so that I may continue to grow in my recovery. Help me continue to remain open-minded to new information. Amen

June 27

Thought for the day
Real joy comes not from ease or riches or from the praise of men, but from doing something worthwhile.

W.T. Grenfell

Meditation
Since beginning my treatment of depression, I have participated in a number of support groups in my community. There I have met some of the most wonderful, helpful, caring people in the world. We share a common bond and understanding of the pain and suffering that we each have been through. We learn how to look after one another. I often speak of the person who first convinced me to seek and accept treatment for my illness. In my opinion, he saved my life. We have developed a friendship over the years in which I truly cherish. As our friendship has grown, I have learned that unlike the early days when I didn't have much support to offer, today he needs me as much as I need him. I became accustomed to calling him and talking solely about my problems and concerns. Then one day, I received a call from him, and this time he needed me to listen to his problems. I remember thinking how unfairly I had placed him on a pedestal, because I felt uncomfortable with the idea that my main source of support was showing signs of weakness. But after I worked through my initial discomfort, I quickly realized how lucky I was to be part of such an awesome circle of support. To be able to be there for my friend, the man who saved my life, was a fantastic feeling. No matter what else is happening in my life today, I can still do something worthwhile by helping someone that is in need of support.

Prayer
God thank you for my friends in recovery. Thank you for putting me in a position that allows me to do something that is truly worthwhile today. Help me never to become so busy that I no longer have time to help others. Amen

June 28

Thought for the day
Recovery is…enjoying life more and enduring it less.
Peggy Katherine Joseph

Meditation
I did not defy my fears and reach out for help, only to endure life. I took a giant leap of faith because I no longer wanted to endure the suffering and humiliation that I had been experiencing for years. My recovery, despite all of its ups and downs, has truly been an experiment about enjoying life. I am still often afraid to try new things out of fear of failure because, prior to recovery, failure had such devastating consequences. But with the help of understanding people, I am now able to look past my fears of failure, and go for it! For me to enjoy my life, I have to be living it to its fullest potential. Today that means taking healthy risks and enjoying the taste of the spices of life.

Prayer
God, today I want to live my life to it's fullest potential. I do not want my fears to exclude me from any healthy adventures that you may have in store for me. Amen

June 29

Thought for the day
Fear is static that prevents me from hearing myself.

Samuel Butler

Meditation
When I am in the deepest, darkest, depths of my depression, I am afraid to live, yet I am afraid to die. Fear is a close, constant companion when I am suffering in the black hole of despair. Today I have learned that my fears and feelings are not necessarily based on fact, especially when I am depressed. My recovery process includes being able to recognize and dispute the static that depression and fear play in my mind. Prior to reaching out and getting the help that I needed, I was unable to do much with the static and disruption that was interfering with my ability to fine-tune my thoughts. Through my recovery, I have learned that with the help of other people, who also suffer from this malady, I can identify my fears and then remove the static from my mind.

Prayer
God, please grant me the insight to identify my fears and, with the help of my friends in recovery, remove the static from my thoughts. Amen

June 30

Thought for the day
Look not mournfully into the Past. It comes not back again.
Wisely improve the Present. It is thine.
Henry Wadsworth Longfellow

Meditation
I have lost years of my life to untreated depression. Lost opportunities and cherished moments with my family and friends have vanished. I cannot recapture that lost time no matter how hard I try. It is now part of my history. I can become very emotional when I consider the price that I have paid. It is very high, and I know that I am not alone in this regard. We who suffer from this illness know the pain of lost moments and opportunities. How do we forgive ourselves? How do we forgive our life? When I feel myself getting angry about the past, I have to go straight to the realization that I was suffering from an illness all those years without any knowledge of it. By accepting and acknowledging my illness, I am able to forgive myself for all the wasted time. I can then make a decision to live today to its fullest. By having a place to go with my depression, I can improve on the present and no longer mournfully wallow in the past.

Prayer
God, help me use my memories as a standard by which I can now measure my personal growth. Do not allow me to beat myself up over the lost time and personal failures. Let me use my experiences as an example to others and myself of how not to live. Amen

July 1

Thought for the day
Loneliness is the first thing which God's eye nam'd not good.

John Milton

Meditation
The disease of clinical depression is a disease of isolation and loneliness. When I am depressed, I no longer want to be around people. Recently I suffered through a short-lived bout with this illness. I noticed that I was embarrassed by my behavior and my thinking to the point that I could not look people in the eye. My friends would call me on the phone to see how I was doing, and at first, I would say fine. I felt like I was doing something wrong and I should be ashamed of myself. Consequently, I wanted to hide from the world. We all know how absolutely horrible it feels to be suffering from this illness only to cut ourselves off from the rest of the world because we feel ashamed. It is at this moment that we must get honest with ourselves and a friend or doctor about what is really going on within us. I had to get around my support and talk about how I was feeling, and as a result, I believe I was able to get the affirmations that I needed to make my last bout shorter than it would have been had I not reached out for help.

Prayer
God thank you for the wonderful people you have put in my life. Help me always feel safe enough to talk with my friends and doctor about how I am really feeling inside. Amen

July 2

Thought for the day
This above all: To thine own self be true.

William Shakespeare

Meditation
I neglected myself for so many years by believing the lies of depression. I suffered so many lost moments by being deceived by this tragic illness. For years, the "old tapes" of depression kept playing and playing in my mind. No matter how hard I tried to convince myself that I was a valuable, worthwhile person, this illness repeatedly told me otherwise. The idea of "to thine own self be true" seemed completely unobtainable because I did not believe I was worth enough to be true to. I just didn't matter any more. Today, by the grace of God and the help of some awesome people, I am practicing, day by day, how to be true to myself. The greatest opportunity for success is contingent on my continuous efforts to hold my depression in remission. I have learned that I cannot always do this with my own resources. I will need help.

Prayer
God, help me always to be true to myself. Please grant me the honesty and insight I will need to continue on this wonderful road of recovery. Amen

July 3

Thought for the day
Friendship is a sheltering tree.
Samuel Taylor Coleridge

Meditation
When I am depressed, my mind and mouth will ambush my heart and soul, and then turn venomously on the people that I love. The constraining feeling that I get when I am unable to speak from my heart is exhausting. The frustration I experience when I am striking out and pushing away rather than asking to be held and loved is wicked and twisted. I need friendship today. I need friendship most when I believe I deserve it least. My experiences in recovery have taught me that friendship is a sheltering tree when the storm clouds of depression appear to be approaching. Despite my many personal testimonies to support this claim, when I do become depressed, I can easily shrug off my past experiences of successfully treating my ailments as "dumb luck" and conclude that "this time" I'm all alone. That is usually when one of my loving brothers or sisters in recovery will cast their umbrella of friendship upon me and keep me safe until the storm of depression subsides.

Prayer
God thank you for the support and friendship I have in my life today. Please help all who are suffering and alone with this illness find the friendship and support they will need to begin their own recovery process. Help us all remember how important it is for us to be friends to one another. Amen

July 4

Thought for the day
I've been so lost I must confess
I've had my share of loneliness.

Aerosmith

Meditation
Time after time in my life, I've been in rooms packed with people, and I've felt completely alone. I've felt like an island in a vast sea of humanity. There were periods when the fear and self-loathing became so intense that they overpowered all rational thoughts and actions. I would sit and stare out the window, or, in the worst case scenario, lie on my bed or on the couch, with the phone off the hook, totally paralyzed. I was a prisoner to my fears, whether imagined or real.

Prayer
God, please remove the fear that is swallowing my very soul. Please help me to rise and move toward the sunlight of your spirit. Amen

July 5

Thought for the day
The truth shall make you free.
John 8:32

Meditation
Much has been written about the persistent pessimism and deceptiveness of depression. We who have suffered from this disease are familiar with how subtly our perception of reality can become warped by this illness. Left untreated, clinical depression can leave us to live our entire lives under illusions of what is real. Recovery is about finding out the true nature of our condition, treating the symptoms of our illness, and then proceeding to live a life free from the confines of warped perceptions and delusional thinking. Today I enjoy an incredible freedom that I have never known before. When I am slipping into the black hole, I am now able to recognize that I am suffering from an illness and not a series of character defects. I am able to stop my frantic search for reasons as to why I feel so terrible and just focus on overcoming the symptoms of this illness by refuting the negative thoughts about myself and replacing them with positive, truthful thinking.

Prayer
God, today please keep me free from the confines of negative, depressive thinking. Grant me the courage to refute all untruthful messages I might attempt to tell myself. Amen

July 6

Thought for the day
The battle, sir, is not to the strong alone; it is to the vigilant.

Patrick Henry

Meditation
Although you may feel certain that you are the weakest of the weak, it takes enormous amounts of strength to persevere against this illness called depression. The battle my friend, is yours, but not yours alone. We will fight beside you every step of the way. Your strength allows you to engage and fight, but your strength alone will never resolve this war between your ears. You're outnumbered and you don't have the weaponry to defeat this enemy. You need allies who will stand vigilant and guard your flanks against surprise attacks. You need to acquire some modern tactics to out maneuver this devious foe. You need to locate some big guns that will be ready when you are lost in the trenches of the black hole and signal for fire support. You must become vigilant yourself, always training and preparing yourself for the next surprise attack.

Prayer
God, help me remain vigilant today, guarding myself against the surprise attacks of depression. Help me always be available whenever anyone calls out for support. Amen

July 7

Thought for the day
Forgive all who have offended you, not for them, but for yourself.

Harriet Uts Nelson

Meditation
When I feel as through I have been the victim of an injustice, I will usually come out of my corner swinging. Filled with self-righteousness and rage, I will quickly pounce on any person or principle that I believe to be threatening or offending. To say I don't enjoy this sort of spirited engagement in verbal warfare every now and then would be less then honest. The problem is I never know when to let it go and move on with life. When I am in the early stages of depression, I will recall all these past offenses and re-live them over and over in my mind, making myself enraged all over again. I then will use these painful experiences as justification to cause myself harm. Pretty sick thinking, wouldn't you say? Yet many of us who suffer from this illness can relate to this insanity. Today it is so important for me to take a good look at my anger when it appears in my life. It may be a warning sign that I am soon going to experience another period of depression in my life. I need to be talking with people in my circle of support about experiences that have me all worked up, regardless of whether they are past, present, or future events. Today I need to get over my anger and resentments as quickly as possible.

Prayer
God, help us today to notice all the warning signs of depression. Help us understand when we are suffering from depression, things are usually not as bad as we make them out to be. Help us realize that anger and resentment, more often than not, are usually masks for what is really ailing us. Amen

July 8

Thought for the day
Courage is doing what you are afraid to do. There can be no courage without fear.

P. Hayes

Meditation
I had become engulfed by my fears. I became afraid to be around people, to answer the phone, or to open my mail. I was slowly losing touch with reality. I had become a prisoner in a self -imposed exile. I was the judge, jury and executioner. The gallows were looking like an option. It got to the point where there were only two alternatives, either take my life or ask for help. Up until this point, even though I had thought of various ways to end it, I had been too afraid. When the pain became too great and I kept waking up to the horrors of another day, I finally asked God for the strength to seek help. What was truly incredible was the almost immediate whirlwind chain of events that occurred which I could never have orchestrated myself. I have since found that God works in mysterious ways and that He will not intervene until I ask Him to. I have also heard that if God's plan were simple enough for me to understand, then it wouldn't be much of a plan. Today my peace of mind is linked to my conscious contact with God.

Prayer
God, please replace my fear with faith. Please help me to trust in your master plan for my life. Amen

July 9

Thought for the day
Our life always expresses the result of our dominant thoughts.

Soren Kierkegaard

Meditation
What thoughts are dominating your mind right now? What is going to be important to you today? Are you planning on obsessing about a situation over which you have no control? Will you spend this day devising ways to hurt yourself more or will you practice self-love? Will you refute all your negative thoughts, all your abusive self-talk, all the lies of depression, and replace them with realistic, honest, healthy appraisals of yourself? Today, let us all make a commitment to think positively about who we are. Let us work hard toward learning how to change years of abusive thinking by making honest, healthy appraisals of our value to our fellow man. Let us seek each other's companionship so that we may overcome the darkness and stand proudly in the light.

Prayer
God, for so many years my thinking was all messed up. Now as I work hard to live a happy, productive life, I am often plagued by the "old tapes" playing between my ears. Help me continue to replace the old, harmful messages of the past, with new, enlightened thinking. Amen

July 10

Thought for the day
Freedom is the right to choose; the right to create for yourself the alternatives of choice. Without the exercise of choice, a man is not a man but a member, an instrument, a thing.

Archibald MacLeish

Meditation
Before I was diagnosed with clinical depression, I was utterly powerless against the landslide of symptoms that engulfed my entire attitude and outlook upon life. As I became surrounded, then buried alive by this persistent push of pessimism, I deceived myself into believing that the events in my life did merit the level of pain and suffering that I was experiencing. I believed that I chose the music that the piper played, and now it was time for me to pay for it. Unbeknownst to me, of real choices, I had few. The choice I have today is simple. I can either treat my depression or not. If I choose the latter, I will become once again, a prisoner of my own orchestrated pain. If I choose treatment, I open myself up to a world full of freedom and possibility.

Prayer
God, when I am suffering from clinical depression, I do not have much choice as to how I think and feel. Thank you for what I do have; the right to choose to treat my illness today. Amen

July 11

Thought for the day
Be not afraid of life. Believe that life is worth living and your belief will help create the fact.

William James

Meditation
Today, I am not afraid to live nor am I afraid to die. I have accepted that I am going to know a physical death, but my faith is that my spirit will live forever. Convinced that my life is just a short moment in eternity, I want to live today. When I was at my lowest, right before the miracle of recovery occurred in my life, I was simultaneously afraid to live and afraid to die. My fear of dying centered on the finality of death and the uncertainty of what the afterlife held in store for me. My fear of living revolved around my relentless self-contempt. The idea of enduring life, wandering aimlessly through the darkness of despair, always letting people down and never amounting to much of anything, was more burden than I could bear. Unable to muster the courage to take my own life, I lived helplessly, hoping that somebody would notice and pity me. I am so grateful that I do not have to live like that any more. By the grace of God, today I do believe that my life is worth living.

Prayer
God, today I will accept that my life is a precious gift that should be nurtured and cherished. Help me remember that suicide will never be the right answer to any of life's problems. Amen

211

July 12

Thought for the day
Thank God every morning when you get up that you have something to do which must be done, whether you like it or not.

Charles Kingsley

Meditation
I am of the humble opinion that people who suffer from clinical depression are bio-chemically predisposed to a lower threshold of ability to endure the troublesome, sad occurrences that frequently happen in everyday life. If we do not have our depression in remission, our reaction to things that we do not like may appear melodramatic to the common observer. For us, it is simply a matter of not having the chemical make-up in place that will allow us to react in a fashion that would be deemed appropriate by the psychiatric community. By participating in a recovery plan, we are able to stabilize our mood and react to life accordingly. Although it can be difficult, I do try to thank God for all the opportunities that I have in my life, whether I particularly care for them or not. I must remember that some of the neatest rewards of my life have blossomed out of situations that I initially found unpleasant.

Prayer
God, help me be grateful for all the things that I have in my life today. Help me trust in your divine plan for me. Show me how to see the good in things that I may find unpleasant so I may present a spirit and enthusiasm for life that will be pleasing to all who may observe. Amen

July 13

Thought for the day
If you do not find peace in yourself you will never find it anywhere else.

Paula A. Bendry

Meditation
I have learned that my attitude and outlook on life has a large impact on my ability to maintain a peaceful spirit. Through trial and error, I have been taught that outside conditions do not have the power to control my internal reaction unless I empower them to do so. Whether we want to believe it or not, we do have a choice as to how we react to any given circumstance. Consider a friend pulling a practical joke on you. Perhaps you don't find the joke all that amusing, but because it was your friend who pulled it on you, you half-heartedly laugh along. Now what happens if a person who you do not particularly care for tries to pull the same joke on you? Are you not quick to tell this individual how little you enjoy them and their stupid attempt at humor? The joke was identical each time, except for the person who was delivering the punch line. Could you not have reacted the same way on both occasions? Of course you could have, but you did not because you didn't really care for the second person. It is important for me to be honest with myself about these sorts of things. I do have choices today. I can relieve myself of a lot of chaos in my life if I am willing to practice reacting to life in a more peaceful manner.

Prayer
God, please help me practice reacting to my life in a more peaceful matter. Help me remember that I cannot always control the events that occur outside of me, but I can change my reaction to them. Amen

July 14

Thought for the day
Sometimes your Heaven is Hell and you don't know why.

Aerosmith

Meditation
There have been many periods in my life when things are going along swimmingly and then my depression strikes again. There doesn't have to be any particular reason other than the fact that I have a chemical imbalance in my brain. Before I accepted and began to treat my clinical depression, I used to look at feeling depressed for no apparent reason as a flaw in my character. I thought it was a moral issue, when in fact, it was the same as being afflicted with any other disease. I didn't want it and I didn't cause it. But, now that I know that I have it, it is my responsibility to take the steps necessary to treat it. The hardest thing for me to do is to take action. I have learned from past experience that if I don't take action, nothing is going to change. Sometimes the first step in this process is something as simple as getting out of bed and picking up the telephone.

Prayer
God, during the onset of depression, help me inventory the events that are occurring in my life. If nothing is happening that I can change, please help me accept and treat my depression. Amen

July 15

Thought for the day
The lowest ebb is the turn of the tide.

Henry Wadsworth Longfellow

Meditation
How often have we been presumably down for the count,
only to stagger to our feet to fight another round? I can
recall many times in my life when I was certain that I was
receiving my final eight count. My depression, left to its
own devices, will weaken me with a relentless flurry of body
blows, and then try to finish me off with a devastating punch
to the head. Bewildered, I will stumble helplessly across the
canvas of life trying to find the safety of my corner. It is
during these lowest moments of my fight for life that I
become desperately willing to reach out for help. As a
result, I have turned the tide against my depression. I have
lived to fight another day.

Prayer
God, please help all the lost fighters in the world find the
safety of your corner. Help them to turn the tide against their
depression so that they may live to fight another day. Amen

July 16

Thought for the day
The love of God is passionate. He pursues each of us even when we know it not.

William Wordsworth

Meditation
When we are suffering from the bondage of depression, it is very difficult for us to feel God's love. In fact, we usually believe we feel God's scorn and dissatisfaction toward our perceived worthless and useless existence. We needlessly punish ourselves so terribly when we allow our depression to dictate our thoughts and convince us that we have been cut off from the love of our Creator. Today we need to make a conscious effort to reinforce the idea that there is a loving Spirit which cares deeply about us. Even when it feels as though the Spirit of God has abandoned us, we must maintain steadfast faith that He is still available to our hearts. It is important for me to remember that God works through people, for people. That being said, I must not look so much for the flash of bright light, but instead, look for the little lights that shine in other people's souls.

Prayer
God, today I will seek and find your miracles working in my life. I will consider and accept how wonderfully you place people in my life that are willing to be helpful in my times of need. Amen

July 17

Thought for the day
Oh Lord, thou givest us everything, at the price of an effort.

Leonardo da Vinci

Meditation
Depression is one of the most frequently occurring mental illnesses or the "common cold" of psychiatry. In 1996, the Director General of the World Health Organization estimated that 340 million people suffer from mood disorders worldwide. Depression is the second most common mental illness after anxiety, but the most common serious mental illness._http://www.depression-net.com/howcommon.html It is important to remember that we are not alone in our fight against this illness. Millions of people are currently suffering from depression, while millions more are currently treating it. Although depression is the most common serious mental illness, it is also one of the most treatable. God has provided us with all the solutions that we need to effectively combat the symptoms of depression, but the willingness to get help has to come from within.

Prayer
God, today, if I begin to experience the symptoms of depression, I will use the support you have made available to me. Thank you for all the wonderful people that have worked diligently to discover methods to improve the quality of life for those of us who are afflicted with this disease. Amen

July 18

Thought for the day
For as he thinks within himself, so he is.
Proverbs 23:7

Meditation
Recently, a psychologist asked me to read an article entitled
The Power of Self-Talk by Harriet B. Braiker, which
appeared in the December 1989 issue of Psychology Today.
Within this article, I found a thinking challenge that I
thought would be worthwhile to try. The idea was that
periodically throughout the day I was to stop and listen to
exactly what I was saying about myself. After a little
practice, I was able to clear the static and begin to hear my
self-talk. It was not pretty at all! I quickly recognized that
my baseline thought process still consisted of many self-
defeating messages. These messages feed my depression
and my depression feeds these messages. Today I really do
not care which came first, but I am concerned with how I
may rid myself of these habitual negative messages. By
stopping and listening to myself regularly, I am able to catch
and challenge much of my abusive thinking. I believe that,
as the proverb said, how I think within myself will determine
who I am. Our untreated depression has left the scars of
negative self-talk within our minds. Our recovery must
include challenging and changing our old abusive ways of
thinking.

Prayer
God, help me to practice listening to my self-talk
periodically throughout the day. Allow me the insight to
discover how my negative thinking has hurt me. Please
grant me the wisdom to replace these thoughts with positive
ones. Amen

July 19

Thought for the day
We cannot do everything at once, but we can do something at once.

Calvin Coolidge

Meditation
I believe that I subconsciously sense the onslaught of depression and instinctively react by attempting desperately to accomplish a multitude of tasks in the hope of shoring up my self-worth. As I begin to slip deeper into my abyss, I compulsively embark on an unavailing search for any person, place, or thing that will make me feel worthwhile. Because I am in such turmoil, I never stay in any one place long enough to possibly gain from it. My experiences have taught me that this is not a very effective method to treat clinical depression. We all have the capacity to do something...but we must accept that we cannot do everything. When we are suffering from depression, it is important to not try to do too much. It is best to focus on the small, simple things that can be accomplished, rather than setting ourselves up for failure by biting off more than we can chew.

Prayer
God, help me not to fall into the trap of my "old tapes" when I am depressed. Help me to remember that it is best for me to stay focused on the small, simple tasks that I can accomplish, rather than attempting to take on more than I can possibly handle. Amen

July 20

Thought for the day
The man who makes no mistakes does not usually make anything.

Edward Phelps

Meditation
Fear of failure has the power to control our lives. When we are depressed, we beat ourselves up over the mistakes we made in the past. Of our legitimate mistakes, we magnify and exaggerate the negative impact that they had on our lives. We begin to believe that we cannot do anything right so we give into the notion that there is no sense in even trying. Leaving our depression untreated, convincing ourselves that it is not real, we rob our families and ourselves of the many joys and rewards that are achieved by trying and succeeding. Today we must ward off complacency and maintain our recovery process. We must not allow this illness to deny us of the life that we truly deserve.

Prayer
God thank you for the rewards that I have been able to reap as a direct result of treating my depression. Help me to remain vigilant against complacency so that I may continue along this joyful path. Amen

July 21

Thought for the day
The hand that holds the whip over our heads is most often our own.

Harvey Eagan

Meditation
An innate characteristic which all of us who are afflicted with clinical depression seem to have in common is the ability to beat ourselves mercilessly. We do not consider for one moment that we are being too hard on ourselves. Despite the appeal from family and friends, we will continue down our path of self-destruction as if it was the only truth in our life. For many of us, this path has become so ingrained into our thinking that, upon beginning recovery, we discover that it can be very difficult at times to change the way we treat ourselves. Today it is important that I continue to develop healthy appraisals of myself. I must practice, using all the resources that are available to me, how to affirm myself on a daily basis.

Prayer
God, help me to practice affirming myself on a daily basis. When I slip into a period of darkness, grant me the wisdom to not be deceived by the lies of this disease. Amen

July 22

Thought for the day
If one advances confidently in the direction of his dreams,
and endeavors to live the life which he has imagined, he will
meet with a success unimagined in common hours.

Henry David Thoreau

Meditation
How do we who suffer from this illness advance confidently
in the direction of our dreams when our dreams have been
shattered so many times? We accept that our depression is
an illness and not a choice. We stop believing that we are
insane, worthless people, and start believing the truth...that
for years our behavior was the result of an illness. As a
result of accepting treatment for this illness, I now have the
freedom to live my life as I choose. I am confident that I can
achieve all that I set out for, as long as I am willing and able
to meet and overcome the challenges along the way.

Prayer
God, I pray for the willingness to continue to place the
necessary effort into my recovery. Help me to use my
abilities today in a matter that is pleasing to you. Amen

July 23

Thought for the day
When I want to understand what is happening today or try to
decide what will happen tomorrow, I look back.

Oliver Wendell Holmes

Meditation
Upon honest self-appraisal, we have to admit that we have
been reacting to our lives inappropriately for many years.
Our undetected depression warped our perceptions of events
to the extent that, when we reflected on our lives, our point
of reference was way off the mark. Today we can use our
past as a vital tool in our recovery. Many times we need to
use our memories to remind ourselves just how far we have
progressed. Other times we use them to see how far we still
have to go. I often find myself comparing how I react to a
problem today to how I reacted in the past. For the most
part, I hope they are not the same. The good news is that our
past does not need to be hidden in the closet. I choose to use
mine as a building block to a bright today and a better
tomorrow.

Prayer
God, help me to benefit from my memories of the past. Help
me to turn a painful time of my life into a positive for my
today and my future. Amen

July 24

Thought for the day
The healthier we become, the less willing we become to
tolerate disaster in our relationships.

Mary Catherine North

Meditation
Untreated clinical depression destroys relationships. It
leaves our spouses feeling empty and confused when their
attempts to recapture the love they had once known never
materializes. All the while we continue to be downtrodden
by an illness that we are not even aware that we have. As we
begin to recover from depression, we may notice that there is
a large vacuum between our spouse and ourselves. They
may be so accustomed to the symptoms of our depression
that it is difficult for them to react to our new outlook on life.
As we progress, we develop new ways to think about
ourselves. Through therapy, we learn how to refute the lies
of our illness and grow to appreciate how well we feel when
we are taking care of ourselves. We begin to expect healthy
reactions from our loved ones. So often the spouse of a
victim of any type of mental illness gets lost in the shuffle.
They suffer too! They need and deserve to receive some
healing also. They need to begin to accept depression as
illness and begin to deprogram their minds of the negative
self-talk. They need to realize that it's not their fault. If you
find yourself in this situation today, schedule some couples
counseling. It is a small investment that yields high returns.

Prayer
God, as I grow in my recovery, please help my spouse to
find the type of support and comfort that I have found. Let
me not forget how great her suffering was during my darkest
hours. Help us to continue to learn how to nurture each other
in a healthy way. Amen

224

July 25

Thought for the day
It is not easy to find happiness in ourselves, and it is not
possible to find it elsewhere.

Agnes Replier

Meditation
Of true happiness, we will know very little if we are not
receiving treatment for our clinical depression. We are
strong willed people. We sometimes struggle to ask for help.
We believe that we should be able to just snap out of our bad
moods and become happy at the drop of a dime. Although
our depression will become very clamorous at times, we
ignore all the warning signs and become more determined to
develop feelings of happiness all on our own. Our denial can
become so great that we lose sight of the fact that we may
not be able to achieve the desired feelings that we had hoped
for. It is amazing how we will repeat the same behaviors
over and over again, each time expecting different results.
We develop a chronic case of the "if onlys" and start to
blame others for our ill feelings. Life becomes very
complicated and exhausting when we attempt to live this
way. When I am suffering from a bout with depression, it is
very important for me to try very hard to relax. I must first
accept that I am experiencing the symptoms of an illness,
then I must call for help. Just as a drowning man, I stand a
much better chance of being saved if I remain calm and stop
fighting the lifeguard who will safely see me to the shore.
Once my bout has subsided, I may continue in my pursuit of
internal peace.

Prayer
God thank you for all the happiness that I have been blessed
with. Help me to remember that I am going to experience

bouts with depression and that these episodes are not an indication that I have failed, but merely symptoms of a treatable illness. Amen

July 26

Thought for the day
No life is so hard that you can't make easier by the way that you take it.

Ellen Glasgow

Meditation
I have been reacting to the problems of my life in a knee-jerk, compulsive manner for so many years that I have to make a conscious effort to remind myself that today I do have a choice as to how I react. I can honestly say that when I exercise that choice, it feels very unfamiliar and awkward. But when I do so, I am very happy with the self-talk that I hear. It is very liberating for me to be able to stop myself from becoming habitually enraged, and react to a situation in a more relaxed, composed manner. I am certain that there are many factors that have contributed to the development of my compulsive way of reacting to life, and I'm sure that my depression definitely added into the equation. Today it is essential to my recovery that I continue to practice taking my life in a more composed, relaxed way. I have to remind myself that it's not what's thrown at me, it's how I catch it that really matters.

Prayer
God, today I will practice reacting to life in a more positive manner. Help me to remember that my problems are minuscule when compared to those who are less fortunate. Amen

July 27

Thought for the day
We don't have time not to have time.

Gary Burke

Meditation
For those of us who have experienced what it feels like to have a gun in our mouth...for those of us who have taken a bottle of pills and fell asleep, only to awaken the next day angry at the world because we were still alive...for those of us who stopped caring about ourselves and commenced to do harmful things hoping that we might die from them...we know first hand that we don't have time not to have time. We know that clinical depression kills people. We know that it is a serious, potentially fatal illness that destroys families and lives. Today we must take our illness seriously. We must guard against complacency and not allow ourselves to isolate from the world. If we are in the black hole, we must call for help. We must rid ourselves of the idea that...if we don't feel better tomorrow we will call a doctor. We must take action right away.

Prayer
God, help all who are suffering from this illness not delay in calling for help. Grant them the courage to reach out of the darkness of despair to find the hands of support that surround them. Amen

July 28

Thought for the day
I was so sick and tired of livin' a lie I was wishin' that I would die

Aerosmith

Meditation
Before I began to treat my clinical depression, I would lie in bed for weeks at a time, trying to sleep my life away. I would use all sorts of different excuses why I couldn't be at work or why I couldn't see my friends of family. I'd say I had the flu, a headache, or I was too tired, when the real reason was that I was suffering from depression. The end result of telling all these lies was that my life would become extremely unmanageable. I would get in trouble for missing work. Then my bills would be late because of not getting paid. This in turn ignited my fears. By isolating myself from my friends, loneliness would overwhelm me. I don't have to tell those lies today. I have to surround myself with safe people who understand my depression and know me well enough to recognize it. I need to get honest with them when I feel the onset of my depression and tell them what I'm thinking and feeling so that they can help me to overcome it.

Prayer
God, please help me to recognize my depression. Please help me to be honest about what is really going on in my life and to ask for help if I need it. Amen

July 29

Thought for the day
Pain is short, and joy is eternal.
Johann Schiller

Meditation
I have never been able to find the words that can accurately describe the pain I was in prior to being diagnosed with clinical depression. I know that at the time I felt utterly hopeless. I cannot explain why some of us have to sink to darker depths then others before we will ask for help. I cannot explain why some of us die from this disease. Pain was my motivator when I attempted to take my own life on numerous occasions. It also turned out to be the motivator that prompted me to talk openly with a doctor about how I was feeling. Today I use my painful feelings and experiences as warning signs that a period of depression may be on my horizon. I can benefit from pain when I accept that it does not have to be a permanent fixture in my life; that I can learn from it and achieve spiritual growth from it if only I allow myself.

Prayer
God, today I will look upon my painful past as evidence of my personal growth. I will use painful experiences as opportunities to reflect on exactly what is happening in my life at any given moment. I will remember that my pain will pass if I work toward that end. Amen

July 30

Thought for the day
Blessed are those who can give without remembering and take without forgetting.

Melvin Schleeds

Meditation
We become extremely needy people when we are suffering from untreated clinical depression. Like the blind man confined to a wheelchair that sits helplessly on a dirty street corner rattling a quarter in a dented soup can, we hopelessly await any type of charity that may come our way. The irony is that if a charitable person does offer us some help, we will tell them to leave us alone as we quickly scurry off into the darkness. As we begin to recover from depression, we may find ourselves reverting back to our patterns of needful behavior whenever we begin to feel a little uncertain about ourselves. One of the most effective ways I have found to break myself of this unhealthy practice is to look for an opportunity to give of myself. I have been taking long enough. Not always by choice, but still the same, it has always been about me. Today it is best for me to see if I can be supportive of somebody else, especially when I am feeling needful. It is amazing how my needs seem to be met whenever I get out of myself long enough to see how somebody else is doing.

Prayer
God thank you for the opportunity to be able to help another human being. Help me to remember that I always have something to give of myself that may be greatly appreciated and make a difference in somebody's life. Amen

July 31

Thought for the day
Comparisons are odious.

John Fortesque

Meditation
Is it hateful and offensive for me to compare myself to others? As a person who has been beaten down from depression and who struggles to maintain a healthy self-esteem, to draw comparisons is probably a form of self-abuse. When I am depressed, I develop the misconception that the rest of the world is happy and I am the only person who is missing out on the fun. I begin to pick myself apart, piece by piece, with the certainty that I will find nothing of value. We can always find somebody who looks better or appears happier. It is easy to find people that seem to be much better off then we are. But if we are going to make that comparison, then we have to be willing to look at the flip side of the coin, which is that there are plenty of people who we would not wish to trade places with. Today the safest comparisons for me to make are the ones that compare me to me. I need to be less concerned with how I measure up against others and more concerned with how I measure up to me. Where growth is evident, I need to congratulate myself. Where I see a legitimate shortcoming, I need to correct it. By staying out of the comparison trap, we stand a much better chance of living within our own skin.

Prayer
God, please help me today not to fall into the comparison trap. Help me to be less concerned with other people's outward appearances and more concerned with my internal condition. Amen

August 1

Thought for the day
Others will mostly treat you the way you treat yourself.
Muhamed Moussa

Meditation
If this was an absolute truth most of us would have been murdered long ago! God knows that we don't treat ourselves very well when we are suffering in the darkness of the black hole. We can become so deflated of life that we just want to lie down in the middle of the road, hoping that somebody will come along and run us over. We become doormats for the world to wipe its muddy boots on, or so it seems to us. Fortunately, we were never able to convince anybody else to do our dirty work. I know it can be painful to reflect on how pitiful we really were, but by doing so, I reinforce my resolve to treat this illness "one day at a time" for the rest of my life. Today we can take care of ourselves. We can treat ourselves with compassion, dignity and respect, and rightfully expect nothing less from everyone we have contact with.

Prayer
God, help me to continue to practice treating myself with compassion, dignity and respect. Please grant me the courage to never accept behavior that is anything less than acceptable to me. Amen

August 2

Thought for the day
I am an old man and have known many troubles, but most of
them never happened.

Mark Twain

Meditation
Depression warps and twists our perceptions of reality so
badly that we develop presumptuous resentments toward the
entire universe while we plummet deeper into a frenzy of
despair. We get ourselves all worked up over tiny,
insignificant events or comments, and then use them as our
basis for self-destruction. If it is brought to our attention
how stupid we appear, we fly off the handle and rage terribly
at the individual who had the nerve to challenge our
reasoning. This sounds funny to me today, but there was a
time when I wasn't laughing one bit. I describe this illness
as hideous. Think of how many years you lived with this
insanity in your life. Consider how grateful you are to be
finally doing something to treat your depression. Think of
the desperate heart that will blow his or her head off tonight
because they just can't take it any longer. Do we have a
responsibility today? You better believe it! If we all work
together, we can bring our fellow sufferers out of the
darkness and into the light. If you don't know how to reach
those who will die from this illness, start a support group in
your neighborhood. Advertise the meeting in your local
newspaper. You will be amazed.

Prayer
God, there are many people who are dying from this illness
and don't even realize it. Please help all of us who are
recovering from this illness reach out to the desperate soul
who needs our help. Amen

August 3

Thought for the day
Life is not war, and people are not the enemy.

Anonymous

Meditation
Many of us who have endured the hardships of depression understand firsthand what it feels like to merely survive life. We feel as though we are in constant battle with the world and that everyone is our enemy. I cannot count how many times I have convinced myself that my life was not worth the effort, and even if it was, I no longer had the will to fight for it. Today we no longer have to fight life or the people in our lives. We can accept that our depression is a real illness and that the messages it tells us about life are false. We can begin to realize that all those people that we blamed for our ill feelings were innocent bystanders, and most importantly, we can begin the process of letting ourselves off the hook.

Prayer
God, today I will work hard to treat myself in a compassionate manner. I will not fight life or the people that are in it. I will accept my depression as a treatable illness. Amen

August 4

Thought for the day
The easiest person to deceive is one's own self.

Edward Bulwer-Lytton

Meditation
Today we live in a society that puts such a high emphasis on being the best; number one! We learned, at a very young age, how to cover-up our imperfections and assume personas that are not genuine. We learn how to be all people at all times. We become chameleons. After years of wearing costumes, it can be very difficult to unmask. If we do, we usually do not know the individual that suddenly appears in our mirror. They look vaguely familiar, but they also look vulnerable and scared. Many of us don't like what we see at all, so we quickly put our disguises back on. Yet that person underneath wants to be seen and heard. They want to tell the world that they have been there the whole time. They want to say that all the other images and behaviors were lies. They want to apologize for the masks' past behaviors. How powerful are these masks? They have the power to suffocate and kill. Our depression becomes a mask. It is a disguise that gets thrown upon us, one that we didn't ask for, and one that we can't remove. We need help removing it from our bodies. It clings heavily to our skin and sends its needles into our minds. It causes us to walk slumped over with our eyes to the ground. It scares away our friends. Thank God we do not have to live like this today.

Prayer
God, help me to stay out of the pitfall of denial and learn to be myself. Today, please grant me the serenity to live within my own skin. Amen

August 5

Thought for the day
Fatigue makes cowards of us all.
Vince Lombardi

Meditation
Our depression can deny us of the willingness to take care of ourselves properly. When we are depressed, we either sleep too much or not at all. Both are considered symptoms and should be looked upon as "red flags" to call your doctor. When we become extremely fatigued, it is very difficult to maintain a positive outlook. We lose interest in our daily living requirements and begin to isolate ourselves from the world. If we sleep too much, the same isolation is occurring. I can recall a time when I would take six-hour naps. I could not understand why I was so tired. Today I know that I was depressed and using sleep as a method to hide from life. I know individuals who, prior to getting help, actually became bedridden for over a month. We must keep a constant watch for the warning signs that appear in the lives of our friends and also in our own. It is detrimental to our recovery to allow anything to make cowards out of us.

Prayer
God, today I will take care of myself properly. I will eat, sleep, think, and feel in an appropriate manner. I will care about myself. If I become extremely depressed, I will ultimately love myself by calling for help and support. Thank you for this day to practice these things. Amen

August 6

Thought for the day
Some circumstantial evidence is very strong, as when you
find a trout in the milk.

Henry David Thoreau

Meditation
If you spend most of your waking moments crying at your
funeral...you might suffer from depression. If you have
been frustrated because you just can't find the right words to
capture the essence of despair that you want to express in
your suicide note...you might suffer from depression. If you
can't decide between lethal injection, hanging, electrocution,
drowning, gunshot, carbon monoxide poisoning, or
plummeting off a tall building to your catastrophic end...you
might suffer from depression. If you find a trout in your
milk...then you've got other problems.

Prayer
God, sometimes when I am depressed I am the last person to
realize it. Depression can creep up and overtake me without
my knowledge if I am not maintaining constant vigilance.
Help me not to grow complacent, but to maintain a faithful
watch for any warning signs that may appear on my horizon.
Amen

August 7

Thought for the day
To affirm life is to deepen, to make more inward, and to exalt the will to live.

Albert Schweitzer

Meditation
For many years I placed the value of my life in the hands of the material world. Life meant achievement and possession. The more I had, the better life was. As my depression progressed, my need for "success" accelerated. I ran as fast as I could, trying to keep the pace. But I just couldn't keep up any longer. When I finally collapsed, I watched as my life left me behind. I was certain this was the end. Convinced that there was nothing left to do but die, I didn't get up. I just wallowed in the gutter of hopelessness and despair, killing my pain and myself with anything that I could find. I had been stripped of my will to fight for my life. As I continued in my dark, downward spiral, the depths of my soul began screaming for help. By the grace of God, the screams were finally heard. Today my life is an inward, upward spiral of affirmation that life is worth living.

Prayer
God thank you for the many opportunities for spiritual growth that my recovery has afforded me. Thank you for the ability to share my experience, strength, and hope with others who also suffer. Amen

August 8

Thought for the day
Give a little love to a child and you get a great deal back.

John Ruskin

Meditation
We are all children of God and we have a right to be here. We have a right to love and to be loved. No matter what shattered past we may have behind us, we have a right to renew and rebuild ourselves in a new light. We no longer have to live in the dark shadows of despair hoping that we will go unnoticed. We can stand firmly in a new belief – a belief that we have suffered from an illness called depression. Today we can love one another without any fear of becoming a victim. If somebody does wrong us, we can accept that they are spiritually sick individuals who have actually wronged themselves by walking an unfaithful walk. Today we can love one another unconditionally. Rid yourself of the shame that this illness has burdened you with. Look in the mirror and tell yourself that you are important today. Tell yourself that you are not all those rotten things that your illness has been saying about you. Feel the love of God in your heart. Love somebody today. Start with the person in the mirror.

Prayer
God, when I become lost in the darkness, please send your helpers to guide me toward the light. Help me to feel your presence in my life. Remind me to affirm myself daily by realizing that I am part of your awesome creation and that I do have a right to be here. Amen

August 9

Thought for the day
He has the right to criticize who has the heart to help.

Abraham Lincoln

Meditation
When I am in the black hole, I become very critical of other people. Nobody, including myself, appears to be able to do anything right. Yet it seems as though I am unable to do anything to improve upon the conditions that I find so appalling. Depression, left unchecked, will bind us up with feelings of uselessness and hopelessness. When we are in this frame of mind, it is so difficult to do anything constructive that might help to better our outlook on life. Today, as a result of seeking and receiving treatment for this illness, we better understand the symptoms and messages that are associated with it. When we find ourselves being unreasonably critical of others, we are able to quickly accept that the problem lies within us. Remember that when you are depressed, your perception of reality becomes so distorted that it cannot be trusted. It has meant a great deal to the quality of my life to be able to become less critical of others, and to accept that my feelings of discontentment may in fact be the result of my illness. That is not to say that this is always the case, but my experience has taught me that I am able to very often free myself from a critical heart, when I consider, in a new light, how and why I am feeling judgmental. By doing so, I am in a much better frame of mind to possibly become helpful rather than a hindrance.

Prayer
God, please free me from the woes of a critical, hindering heart. Help me to quickly sort though any distorted thinking that may stand in my way of becoming helpful to others. Amen

August 10

Thought for the day
Let us then be up and doing,
With a heart for any fate,
Still achieving, still pursuing,
Learn to labor and to wait.

Henry Wadsworth Longfellow

Meditation
The waiting is the hardest part. I consider my life today to be nothing short of a miracle. I went through hell to get to where I am today, so I quickly take exception to any person, place, or thing that threatens the stability in my life that I have grown to treasure. When I relapse into a period of depression, I know what I have to do to take care of myself. I'm no longer willing to tolerate this illness destroying my life, so I am willing to do whatever it takes to relieve myself of its symptoms. Sometimes I forget that my willingness alone will not make the feelings go away. There is a process involved...a process that occasionally requires more time and effort than I was anticipating. Whenever I see my doctor and she suggests changing medication, I usually experience feelings of defeat and failure, as if I had something to do with it. We all know that the effects of medications sometimes take up to two weeks to develop. This is the time that I must remember to labor and wait. It is very important for me to remain in close contact with my support group and, if necessary, my doctor. By repeatedly pulling through past bouts with depression, I know that my suffering will eventually subside and I will be able to continue along with my life as happily as I was before.

Prayer
God thank you for seeing me through so many down times in my life. Help me to remember and prepare for my next bout with depression. Amen

August 11

Thought for the day
The worst loneliness is not to be comfortable with yourself.

Mark Twain

Meditation
After years of living with abusive, self-destructive self-talk, what messages are you saying about yourself today? Do you like the person that you see in the mirror each morning, or do you still struggle to look yourself in the eye? Are you still afraid to be alone with your own thoughts? Do you live each day with feelings of impending doom? Depression has a way of isolating us from people, while filling us with thoughts of self-hatred and despair. Really, the worst loneliness is to hate yourself. Today we must continue to take steps toward learning to live comfortably within our own skins. We must aggressively refute the lies of this illness while affirming that we are worthy companions to others and ourselves.

Prayer
God, today I will affirm to myself that I am a worthy companion to others and myself. I will remind myself that the disease of depression has a way of isolating me from other people. Today, I will remember that I must exercise a plan of preventive maintenance in my life. Amen

August 12

Thought for the day
Recovery is a civil war, but it is a war that can be won.

Sister Imelda

Meditation
We can consider each bout with depression as a battle within our internal civil war. Some battles are won overwhelmingly. Others are a little more drawn out and take a greater toll on our defenses. Yet others are intense hand to hand combat in the trenches of our mind. Sometimes it may feel as if we have lost, when in all actuality, the outcome was a draw. I have accepted that I am fighting for my life. I understand that this civil war of mine will not be completely won until it is my time to pass on. I am prepared for the many skirmishes that I may have to endure throughout the rest of my life.

Prayer
God, grant me the courage and the endurance to fight the good fight so that I may live another day to prepare myself spiritually for the moment that you say I no longer have to fight. Amen

August 13

Thought for the day
Henceforth I ask not good fortune, I myself am good fortune.
Walt Whitman

Meditation
Today, whether we are depressed or not, we can consider ourselves "good fortune" because we have accepted that we suffer from a treatable illness and have begun to do something about it. We no longer have to hope that something will come our way to make us feel better. We don't have to exhaustively attempt to manipulate and control people or circumstances any more. Henceforth, we may move forward with our heads held high, with the knowledge that we are not the pitiful, worthless creatures we once thought. Today we are "good fortune".

Prayer
God, thank you for the wisdom I now have in regard to clinical depression. Thank you for the teachings I have received that have shown me that I am not my negative self-talk but rather "good fortune". Amen

August 14

Thought for the day
Let us run with patience the race that is set before us.

Hebrews 12:1

Meditation
Part of my recovery process has been accepting the things I cannot change in my life. I have wasted a great deal of time and energy trying to change the circumstances of my life that I have found disturbing, while never considering that I was going about it all wrong. At some point I had to become willing to be honest with myself long enough to understand that I was running in the wrong race. Today, I fully accept the fact that I suffer from a treatable, yet potentially fatal illness called depression. I understand that I may never rid myself of this malady, that the best I may hope for is a daily reprieve that is contingent on my treatment efforts.

Prayer
God, help me to remember that I may have to treat my depression periodically for the rest of my life. Help me to accept that I do suffer from this illness, but remind me that there is much that I can do about it today. Amen

August 15

Thought for the day
Success is to be measured not so much by the position that one has reached in life as by the obstacles which he has overcome while trying to succeed.

Booker T. Washington

Meditation
I find it very difficult to acknowledge and reward myself for the many obstacles that I have overcome in my life. It is very easy for me to discredit my efforts as "dumb luck" without giving any serious consideration as to how much hard work actually went into reaching of my goals. So often we take our progress in recovery for granted. Every so often it is good for us to reflect upon how hopeless we felt prior to receiving treatment for our depression. We should remember how lost and alone we were. We should recall how certain we were that suicide was our only option. Today we can feel good about taking responsibility for ourselves by treating our depression. It was by no means a small task for us to get where we are today. We may rejoice that we are successfully treating this illness one day at a time.

Prayer
God, help me to affirm myself today. Help me to acknowledge that by treating my depression one day at a time, I am a success. Amen

August 16

Thought for the day
Only those who dare to fail greatly can ever achieve greatly.
Robert F. Kennedy

Meditation
I am amazed by the rationalizations many of us will cling to when it comes to taking anti-depressant medications. Here we are, teetering on the verge of suicide, when a doctor diagnoses us with depression. Bear in mind that we have not been able to put together two positive thoughts for months, and we can't keep the shotgun out of our mouths, yet we are worried about "how the medication might make us feel". This sort of thinking offers further evidence that untreated depression will distort our perceptions of reality to the point that we may no longer have the ability to help ourselves. Many of us have been in this place. We all know how scary it can be to surrender to a new idea. Our fear of failure has helped to keep us in the darkness of despair for many years. Then, by the grace of God, we dared to "fail greatly" by accepting help. We pushed aside our fear of treatment or medication not working for us, and we decided to give it a try. Today we can agree that the life we know outside of the darkness is one of our greatest achievements.

Prayer
God, grant me the courage to overcome all my fears that may be holding me back from achieving healthy, enriching experiences in my life. Amen

August 17

Thought for the day
A body seriously out of equilibrium, either with itself or with it's environment, perishes outright. Not a mind. Madness and suffering can set themselves no limit.

George Santayana

Meditation
When my depression set in, I felt shipwrecked in a vast sea of humanity. I was constantly trying to row against the current. As I drifted further and further off course, family and friends began to look like tiny grains of sand on a far off beach. I steered aimlessly in circles, trying to keep the tidal wave of life from crashing down upon me. As I approached what I thought to be the safety of an island, it would always turn out to be only a mirage. I no longer knew what was real or what was make believe. Was I losing my mind? I found the answer to that question was no. I might have been insane at that time, but I was suffering from clinical depression. It was caused by a chemical imbalance in my brain. My body was no longer producing enough of the "feel good" chemicals. And, yes, it could be arrested and treated. Over time I would be able to lead a reasonably happy and contented life. The first step was being referred to a good psychiatrist and psychologist who understood depression. After a period of time we were able to stabilize the roller coaster ride in my mind and later tackle some of the emotional scars that had developed over the years. I realize today that it is just as important to treat the chemical imbalance as it is to treat my insane thinking.

Prayer
God, please lead this wayward soul back on course. Please give me the strength and insight to follow the map that you have placed before me. Amen

August 18

Thought for the day
Ambition can creep as well as soar.
Edmund Burke

Meditation
What are your aspirations for today? Do you plan to leap tall buildings with a single bound? Are you going to rise to the top of the heap and prove yourself worthy to be called the best, or are you just going to focus on not entertaining any suicidal thoughts today? When I am suffering from depression, my ambitions begin to escape me as I creep along in the darkness of my despair. I sometimes sink so deep into the black hole that the only objective I may hope to obtain is to reach out for help...either by calling my doctor or a close friend. Although it may not feel so at the time, my efforts to call for help are very ambitious indeed. By doing so, I quickly begin to crawl out of the darkness and into the light where I can truly discover that I may aspire to be anything that I choose to be.

Prayer
God, help me to acknowledge my small ambitions along with the large. Help me to remember that all my efforts to improve the quality of my life are but building blocks that I may continually build upon. Amen

August 19

Thought for the day
You commit a sin of omission if you do not utilize all the power that is within you. All men have claims on man, and to the man with special talents, this is a very special claim. It is required that a man take part in the actions and clashes of his time than the peril of being judged not to have lived at all.

Oliver Wendell Holmes

Meditation
Today, our recovery empowers us to accomplish many things that we once considered out of reach. As such, we have an inherent responsibility to readily carry the message of hope to all that may presently be in need of support. If I am attending any form of a social gathering, whether it be a church social, school event, or town meeting, I have a responsibility to be watchful and aware of the symptoms of depression. If I happen to overhear an individual talking about how much of a failure they are or witness someone demonstrating despairing behavior, I must overcome my fears of rejection and confrontation, and attempt to help this person. I must also accept that my intrusion may not be welcome and my words may fall on deaf ears, yet I must make the effort. My special claim today is that I have been given an endless supply of seeds that I must be willing to plant whenever and wherever the opportunity may present itself.

Prayer
God, today I will be mindful of other people's behavior. If I notice a neighbor, co-worker, or friend exhibiting the symptoms of depression, I will take the time to discuss and inform them about this illness and the treatments that are now available. Amen

August 20

Thought for the day
You cannot fly like an eagle with the wings of a wren.

William Henry Hudson

Meditation
Today I must not allow my battleship mind to get ahead of my rowboat ass. I must be rigorously honest with myself regarding my abilities and limitations. So often, especially when I am in the early stages of depression, I begin to overburden myself with unachievable goals. As I fall short of the mark, I point to my failure as justification of why I am so depressed. When I get caught up in this "sick dance", the dance of self-sabotage and self-fulfilling prophecies of failure, I am clouding my ability to recognize the true nature of my condition. We all are guilty of this sort of behavior to varying degrees. What is important today is our ability to admit it and our willingness to change. We certainly cannot fly like an eagle with wings of a wren, but we can develop whatever wings we desire if we are willing to exert the necessary effort.

Prayer
God thank you for my willingness to change. Thank you for the faith that I now have, a faith that tells me I can accomplish whatever I desire as long as I remain honest with myself regarding my abilities and limitations. Amen

August 21

Thought for the day
A friend is one before whom I may think aloud.

Ralph Waldo Emerson

Meditation
My friendships prior to recovery were superficial at best. I imagine that was the case out of necessity rather than choice. I just could not identify or express how I was feeling very well, so I associated with people who reacted to life in much the same fashion as I did. Often, recovery is a process of identifying authentic feelings and then expressing them to another human being. For many of us, this process takes years. It can be very frightening to open ourselves up to a person whom we hesitantly have decided to halfway trust. I must tell you though, that by doing so, I probably saved my life. Many of us have denied ourselves relief from depression by lying to our doctors about how we really were feeling. We have pushed away potential friendships because we were afraid that they might "find us out". Today, many of us have found true friendship with each other by sharing a common denominator. By being honest with another person about how we are feeling, we have learned to treasure and hold our friendships in the highest regard.

Prayer
God thank you for the blessings that my friendships have brought into my life. Today, if I slip into a period of depression, I am no longer alone. I have people in my life who I am able to call, friends that understand exactly how I am feeling...friends who have been there themselves. Today I pray that all the lost, depressed souls find the friends that they need. Amen

August 22

Thought for the day
He maketh his sun to rise on the evil and on the good, and sendeth rain on the just and on the unjust.

Jesus Christ

Meditation
Contrary to the belief that many of us have, our depression is not a form of punishment that has been placed upon us by a vengeful Creator. Prior to beginning my recovery, when I was depressed, I would feel ashamed of myself because I appeared to be so ungrateful. I felt as though God probably didn't have much patience for a person that had so much to live for, yet wanted to die. Feeling completely isolated from God and the rest of the world; I proceeded with my life of self-destructive behavior. Today I understand that untreated depression will interfere with my ability to maintain the spiritual condition by which I desire to live my life. I understand God as the Divine Spirit and my Creator, a God who loves me unconditionally.

Prayer
God, today please help me to remember that when I am depressed, I am not worthless and ungrateful, but rather just simply exhibiting the symptoms of a treatable illness. Amen

August 23

Thought for the day
There is nothing so moving – not even acts of love or hate –
as the discovery that one is not alone.

Robert Ardrey

Meditation
Clinical depression manifests itself in our lives in so many
different ways. There are a multitude of warning signs and
as many symptoms, both mental and physical. Beyond
persistent pessimism, I declare isolation as the most
dangerous behavior that is associated with this disease.
When the sadness won't go away, we begin to isolate
ourselves from our employer, family, and friends. We
become filled with self-pity, guilt and shame. We begin to
believe that we are worthless and hopeless. We all know
from our shared experiences, how unbearable the feelings of
loneliness and despair can be. The irony is that we feel all
alone along with an estimated 20 million other Americans. I
cannot express completely, the relief and security that I felt
once I began to meet and talk with people who also suffered
from this illness. I felt liberated knowing that, not only was I
not alone, but that I never have to be alone again.

Prayer
God, I pray today for all people that are currently suffering
from the devastating loneliness of depression. I ask that you
grant them the courage to seek the help and the fellowship
that I have found. Amen

August 24

Thought for the day
You feel the way you do right now because of the thoughts
you are thinking at this moment.

David D. Burns

Meditation
What are you thinking right now? Do your thoughts and
feelings "add up", or does one seem to be out of proportion
with the other? So often when we are depressed, our
feelings don't match our thoughts. We become confused as
to why we feel so sad, because there seems to be nothing that
bad happening in our life. To compensate for this disparity,
we "lower" our thoughts to match our feelings. We do so
out of necessity because, left unbalanced, we can begin to
believe that we are going insane. For years I let my feelings
dictate my thoughts. I never gave any serious consideration
as to whether I could change my thinking or not. Today, if
we are depressed, we must refute our feelings with the facts.
We must not allow ourselves to fall into our old patterns of
thinking by lowering our thoughts to match our ill feelings.
We must recognize the symptoms of our illness and begin
the healing process by allowing ourselves positive
affirmation.

Prayer
God, help me today to refute all negative thoughts and
feelings that I may have. Help me to quickly recognize
when I am depressed so that I may recover to a sound state
of thinking and feeling. Amen

August 25

Thought for the day
My private war has been fought within the trenches of my own mind.

Jeffrey Ross

Meditation
I must remain ever vigilant in my fight against depression. I cannot rely entirely upon my own instinctive actions to recognize and react to an attack. I must surround myself with friends and professionals who, at times, know me better than I know myself. Left to my own devices, my first reaction will be to isolate. The end result of isolation will always be self-destructive thoughts and actions.

Prayer
God, please grant me the willingness to let people get close to me. Please allow me to be open-minded enough to hear them when they tell me that they see the self-destructive process beginning. Amen

August 26

Thought for the day
Nothing is more difficult than competing with a myth.

Francoise Giroud

Meditation
I will liken living with depression to competing with a myth.
This illness causes me to believe things that are not true. It
distorts my ability to see things for what they really are. It
can cause me to appear harsh and extreme while I push away
the people who are trying to help me. It has caused me to
confront the imagined and left me filled with presumptuous
resentments. I was living a lie for so many years that it
angers me to consider what I have lost. There is nothing we
can do to change our history today except to improve each
day, from this day forward. By treating our depression and
helping others, we can create a new history that we can be
proud to claim. By clearing the battlefield that has raged
between our ears for so many years, we can create a playing
field on which we may fairly compete.

Prayer
God, please help and protect me as I continue on my journey
to uncover the truths of my life. Help me to remember that
things are often not as "bad" or "good" as they may appear
on the surface...that a deeper purpose usually can be found
upon closer examination. Amen

August 27

Thought for the day
Think in terms of depletion, not depression...You can understand how a body can replenish itself, whereas it may be difficult to understand the way out of depression.

Claire Weekes

Meditation
I greatly accelerated my ability to help myself once I began to consider some new ways to think about depression. This idea of thinking in terms of "depletion rather than depression" is excellent. It allows me to focus on the biochemical aspects of this illness rather than all the negative messages that bombard me when I am suffering. To simply consider that my deep sadness is caused by a depletion of serotonin in my brain, rather than the actualities of my life is uplifting. To understand there are many fantastic medications that are now available...medications that are suited for increasing the concentration of serotonin in my brain...is liberating. Today I must remain open-minded to new ideology and scientific progress if I hope to continually overcome my occasional bouts with this disease.

Prayer
God, today I understand that the cost of daily remission from clinical depression is constant vigilance. I understand that I must remain open-minded to new ideology and scientific progress if I hope to continually overcome my occasional bouts with this disease. Amen

August 28

Thought for the day
Do not wish to be anything but what you are, and try to be that perfectly.

St. Francis de Sales

Meditation
Today it is important for me to remember that what I am and who I am can be very different. It is equally important for me to accept both realities and try to live each perfectly. My spiritual and moral fiber has designed who I am while what I do defines what I am. My hopes and dreams are part of who I am today, therefore it is important for me to aspire to the continual betterment of my life so that I may soon recognize that for which I once dreamed. The preface to all of this is acceptance. I had to first accept the truths about my mental, physical, and spiritual condition to understand where I was coming from before I could begin to determine where I was heading. I had to accept that I suffered from clinical depression and couldn't expect much improvement in the quality of my life until I began to treat it.

Prayer
God thank you for the awareness that we have been blessed with today. Thank you for the freedom to improve ourselves so that we may fulfill many of our dreams. Amen

August 29

Thought for the day
I have learned to have very modest goals for society and myself, things like clean air, green grass, children with bright eyes, not being pushed around, useful work that suits one's abilities, plain tasty food, and occasional satisfying nookie.

Paul Goodman

Meditation
What a joy it is when we are able, for perhaps the first time in many years, to comfortably sit back and enjoy the simpler pleasures of life. For so long we have been focused on all that is wrong with our life that we have allowed all that is "right" to pass us by. Today I may find great pleasure in knowing that I never have to suffer alone again. I can rejoice in the fact that I now have the tools by which I may build a life that is pleasing to me. I no longer have to accept that which is unacceptable and I no longer have to believe that extravagance and excess will ever fill the voids in my life. I may now focus on the really important things like being a better husband, father, neighbor and friend. Today I can enjoy the rewards of life like clean air, green grass, children with bright eyes, not being pushed around, useful work that suits my abilities, tasty food, and occasional satisfying nookie.

Prayer
God, help me not to chase my illusions of grandeur in the hope that the conquest will somehow make me feel complete. Remind me of the fact that my most peaceful experiences in life have always centered on the simplest of things. Amen

August 30

Thought for the day
I've developed a new philosophy – I only dread one day at a time.

Charles M. Schulz

Meditation
Of course there is obvious humor in today's thought but upon closer examination I find an idea that can aid me when I am depressed. When I am in the black hole I don't dread one day... I dread yesterday, today and tomorrow all at the same time. It would actually be an improvement to my attitude if I were able to just dread one day at a time. Today I do recognize that when I am depressed my condition is only temporary. I understand that I can help to expedite my recovery by seeing my doctor and talking with the understanding friends that are in my circle of support. I have developed a new philosophy regarding my depression – a philosophy that says my depression is a temporary medical condition that can be treated...a condition that exhibits the symptoms of dreadful thoughts. As a result, I know that if I must dread...I only have to dread one day at a time because "this too shall pass".

Prayer
God, please help me practice living one day at a time. So often I can get caught up in worrying about things that are yet to come that I miss the precious "now". Help me to remember that if I must dread, I only have to do so one moment at a time. Amen

August 31

Thought for the day
I have been driven many times to my knees by the overwhelming conviction that I had nowhere else to go. My own wisdom, and that of all about me seemed insufficient for the day.

Abraham Lincoln

Meditation
There have been times in my life, and there will continue to be times in my life, when all there is left for me to do is pray. In the past, it has been during my darkest, most perplexing hours that I have been propelled to fall to my knees and ask my Creator for guidance and inspiration. It is there that I have surrendered to the fact that I could not pull through on my own any longer. Although I occasionally want to scoff, the evidence of my life does indicate that my prayers have been answered...not always the answer that I was searching for, but answered all the same in a matter that was far superior to anything I might have been able to contrive. My wisdom today tells me that it would serve me well to develop an overwhelming conviction to get on my knees and quietly pray for the knowledge of God's will each day of my life, whether I have nowhere else to go or not.

Prayer
God, so often I wait until I am completely overburdened before I turn to you in prayer. Help me to completely accept that the serenity and peace I seek will be found within a prayerful life. Amen

September 1

Thought for the day
I can feel guilty about the past, apprehensive about the future, but only in the present can I act. The ability to be in the present moment is a major component of mental wellness.

Abraham Maslow

Meditation
Learning to live in the moment is perhaps one of the most challenging components of my recovery. When I am depressed, I am usually wallowing in the sorrows of my past. When my depression is in remission, I often find myself spending the majority of my time living in the future. Meanwhile, the "here and now" is happening to me, and I miss out on the joys of the moment because I am busy elsewhere. As with combating our negative self-talk when we are depressed, learning to focus on the moment and live within the present 24-hours requires patience, diligence, and constant vigilance. Today my experience has taught me that it is in the "moment" in which I want to live my life. Worry is worthless and the past is the past. Today is the only day I have. What I make of it is entirely up to me. I no longer want to live my life looking through the rear-view mirror or toward the finish line on the horizon. I want to be able to enjoy what I am doing right now.

Prayer
God, help me to live this day to the fullest. Help me to remember that this is the only day I have to live. The past is the past, and tomorrow is not guaranteed. Please grant me the focus that I will need to break my old patterns of wallowing in the past and worrying about the future so that I may truly rejoice in this day that you have made for me. Amen

September 2

Thought for the day
The point of therapy is to get unhooked, not thrash around on how you got hooked.

Maryanne Walters

Meditation
Many of us treat our depression with a combination of therapy and medication. In therapy we find a safe environment in which we can honestly discuss how we are thinking and feeling about our life. We also might take advantage of the opportunity to revisit some "old skeletons" that have been hanging around in our closets for some time. Some of us have other afflictions that we also need to be treating. Illnesses like alcoholism and chemical dependency must also be addressed if we hope to overcome our struggle with clinical depression. As we dive into some of our more painful memories, we stir up emotions that may make us uncomfortable and perhaps depressed. When I am in this situation, it is very important that I hang in there and trust the process. By doing so, I have learned how to quickly and honestly evaluate situations, and walk away from them with an understanding of how and why they affected me the way they did. Today I consider this a gift. By working hard in therapy, I now have the ability to get unhooked many times over by using these new insights.

Prayer
God thank you for the rewards that I have received as a result of working hard to better myself. Thank you for the courage that I needed to trust this process long enough to begin to reap its benefits. Amen

September 3

Thought for the day
What does not destroy me, makes me strong.

Friedrich Nietzsche

Meditation
A few years ago my untreated depression nearly ended my life. I was certain I would never know a better way to live...I was convinced that it was my time to die. My internal voice was screaming for relief from the persistent push of this disease. My spirit was beaten down so badly that my will to live had become practically nonexistent. By the grace of God I finally saw a doctor regarding my suicidal thoughts. I had no preconceived notions concerning what the outcome of that visit might bring about, but I did know in my heart that I was dangerously close to killing myself. At that time, I had no knowledge of the disease of depression or its related symptoms. Once I was diagnosed, I began to recover my lost life. Today, along with millions of other men and women, I fight against this illness one day at a time. It has not destroyed me; it has made me stronger. I am determined not to die by suicide today. I plan to die with this disease, not from it.

Prayer
God, please give us the courage and strength to continue to fight off the symptoms of this illness...one day at a time. Help us to see how much stronger we are today, by surviving through those darkest times. Amen

September 4

Thought for the day
When a man is wrapped up in himself he makes a pretty small package.

John Ruskin

Meditation
When I am in the darkness, I become a very self-conscious, self-centered person. I don't think there is much unusual or wrong with that. In fact I think it is a natural reaction to protect an open wound. Unfortunately, when I am depressed, all I can think about is how everything that is occurring in my life is affecting me. It becomes difficult for me to have compassion or concern for somebody else because I just feel like dying. Depression can cause us to isolate from our family and friends for long periods of time. We can't help but to become wrapped up in ourselves while we are alone in our self-imposed banishment from life. Everybody suffers when we are in this condition. Today, as a result of treatment, therapy, and faith, I can effectively get out of myself long enough to pick up the phone and call for help if need be. I know that isolation is no good for me when I am depressed. I also know that if I force myself to become aware of the world around me, and make a conscious effort to participate in somebody else's life in some helpful way, I will begin to break out of my very small box.

Prayer
God, help me today to be free from the trap of isolation. Please free me from self-centeredness and help me to practice participating in somebody else's life in some helpful way. Amen

September 5

Thought for the day
No one can make you feel inferior without your consent.
Eleanor Roosevelt

Meditation
Many of us have experienced scorn and disapproval from a family member or friend after they have tried in vain to help us "snap out" of our depressed mood. Exasperated, our spouses may have threatened to end the marriage because they "apparently aren't making us happy any more". Many of us have lost our families already because of our undiagnosed, untreated depression. If you happen to be such a person, you have experienced a tragic loss…but it was not completely your fault! As with alcoholism and chemical dependency, there is still a world of ignorance that surrounds the disease of depression. How responsible we are for our words and deeds while we are unknowingly afflicted is uncertain to me. I do know that once we have been diagnosed, we become 100% responsible to seek and continue to seek the treatment that we need to recover. Part of this process for me has been freeing myself of resentments and forgiving those people who have hurt me…whether out of ignorance or spite. I also must aggressively seek to maintain a positive image of myself by ridding my mind of feelings of inferiority and worthlessness. Today I know that I don't have to feed into negative thinking any longer.

Prayer
God, please grant me the spirit of forgiveness whenever bitterness and resentment enters my life. Please remind me that I no longer have to allow myself to be scorned by anybody…that other people do have the right to be angry and bewildered, but I have the right to disagree. Amen

September 6

Thought for the day
I seem to have an awful lot of people inside me.

Edith Evans

Meditation
When I am depressed and feeling sad because of all the things that I am not, it can be very helpful for me to consider all the things that I am. I have a great friend who will occasionally ask me to write down on a piece of paper all that I am, excluding what I do for a living. Believe it or not, there was a time when I couldn't think of anything to write. Today I know that I am many different things to many different people. Most importantly, I recognize that I am not as worthless as I once imagined. We all wear many different hats, some by choice, others by necessity. Regardless, when we are depressed, it is a natural tendency for us to conclude that we don't wear any of the hats very well and that everyone around us would be much better off if somebody else would start wearing our hats for us. If somebody does step forward and starts to take on our responsibilities, we use that as more evidence to confirm our utter worthlessness to the world. It is important to my recovery today to be honest with myself regarding the many roles I play in life, and to limit those roles in direct proportion to my ability to successfully handle them. I have to accept that when I am depressed, I may have to place some of my activities on hold or ask somebody to help me out.

Prayer
God, I thank you for the full and enriching life that I now know. I have many different roles that I play for many different people, but let me remember the most important role that I play today is the role of recovery. Amen

269

September 7

Thought for the day
A man must learn to forgive himself.
Arthur Davison Ficke

Meditation
At some point in my recovery I had to stop blaming myself for suffering from depression. I have found that forgiving myself is not always easy to accomplish because I have such an ingrained compulsion that demands perfection at all times. Believing I am in control of everything that happens in my life is an imaginary defense against being hurt, but it also means I am responsible for everything that goes wrong. Of course today I recognize there are many things in my life over which I am powerless and therefore not responsible for, but I still on occasion will hold myself accountable for things that were out of my control. Today I must forgive myself of my transgressions only, and no longer assume responsibility for events in which I should not be holding myself accountable.

Prayer
God, you have so graciously forgiven me of my many transgressions, yet I sometimes struggle to forgive myself. Please help me to learn self-forgiveness and bless me with the grace to readily forgive others. Amen

September 8

Thought for the day
The cruelest lies are often told in silence.

Robert Louis Stevenson

Meditation
It is amazing to me to consider how badly I have been hurt by the perpetual lies of my youth...how I matured into adulthood with a set of thoughts about myself that were destructive and untrue. I have exhausted much emotion to uncover my silent lies, perhaps exerting more energy toward discovering the "why" of the lies, instead of implementing my new found truths into my life. It is so easy to stay lost in the sickness of my past. It can become frightening when I consider how distorted and deranged my thinking really was prior to recovery. It is just as scary to consider that I must remain on guard against the cruelest lies I am still able to tell myself when I lock myself away in my own silence. Today it is so important for us to begin to talk about how we are thinking and feeling with somebody we can trust. It is paramount that the people we select, whether professionals or members of our circle of support, are people who will be able to quickly identify our "lies" and help us refute them. I have such people in my life today. They have taught me how to read the underlying messages of life. It is now my experience that these are the only messages that really appear to be worth reading.

Prayer
God thank you for the insight I have received as a result of the wonderful people you have put in my life today. Help me continue using all the resources that you have made available to me so that I may continue my work as a recovering member of my community. Amen

September 9

Thought for the day
The complacent, the self-indulgent, the soft societies are about to be swept away with the debris of history.
John F. Kennedy

Meditation
We are living in a very exciting age...the age of the *Internet*. Despite its growing pains, there is much to be said about the positive impact that it has had on commerce and community. As depression sufferers, it is important that we not isolate from the world when we are experiencing a bout with this serious illness. Some of us are shy, so the idea of reaching out to a total stranger for help can be frightening. But now there are many online communities in which we can participate...communities that we can feel comfortable to talk within...a place where we can get the initial support that we may need to encourage us to call a doctor or a close friend. I often visit the chat rooms that I find on the Internet, and participate in the ongoing discussions. It is a wonderful thing to me, seeing people helping each other out...listening to each other's troubles and pain...sharing experience strength and hope with each other. We truly never have to be alone again if we become willing to participate in all that this life has to offer us.

Prayer
God thank you for the many new discoveries of this century...discoveries that have become powerful resources in the successful treatment of this serious mental illness. Amen

September 10

Thought for the day
We're all of us sentenced to solitary confinement inside our
own skins, for life.

Tennessee Williams

Meditation
What we need to be learning how to do today is how to live
within our own skin comfortably. I imagine confinement in
a small cell with a person I cannot stand. There is no
escaping this person's company, and so we fight terribly
with each other all day long. We are constantly causing each
other physical and mental pain, never ceasing in our devising
of new ways to torment each other. We set each other up by
establishing fraudulent truces, and as soon as the other lets
his guard down...WHAM...we knock'em across the back of
the head. I can easily relate my battles with depression to
this analogy. Today it is important for me to recognize that
when I am angry and feel like I am fighting against the entire
universe, it is usually me who I am really fighting against.
Our recovery is a continual experience of improving self-
esteem so that we may comfortably live within our own skin.

Prayer
God, help me today to do things that will not be harmful to
my self-esteem. Help me continue in my pursuit of inner
peace and goodwill toward my fellow man. Amen

September 11

Thought for the day
What's gone and what's past help
Should be past grief.

Shakespeare, 'The Winter's Tale'

Meditation
One of the more painful components of depression is how I will drudge up painful memories of the past while I am wandering around aimlessly in the darkness of my despair. I will allow myself to feel the same pain and endure the same suffering today as I did when the original sorrow fell upon me perhaps twenty years ago. The danger in this mindset is that as I grow older, I have naturally accumulated more painful memories. The cumulative impact of all my painful experiences of the past is rapidly becoming more than I can sustain. Therefore it is of the utmost importance to my well-being that I continually remain aware of the onslaught of depression and all it entails. Today if I become depressed, I am aware of my patterns of thinking into the past. I am now able to recognize what is happening within me and understand that what's gone and what's past…should be past grief, not to be revisited today.

Prayer
God, please help me today to grieve when appropriate…and then allow the past to remain the past. Help me to recognize that when I'm wallowing in the sorrows of yesterday, it could be a clear indication that I am depressed today. Amen

September 12

Thought for the day
Sorrow is a fruit; God does not allow it to grow on a branch
that is too weak to bear it.

Victor Hugo

Meditation
God knows we have all felt certain that we could not handle
any more sorrow or grief in our lives. Many of us have
crumbled beneath the enormous weight of disparagement,
convinced to a man that we would never be able to rise
again. It troubles me to consider how many people are
suffering alone with this illness right now without the
slightest clue as to what is actually wrong with them...and
that there is plenty of love and support awaiting them if they
could just be reached. God has placed upon us the wisdom
to understand and treat this illness, now we must carry the
message of hope that has been so freely given to us to all that
are still lost in the darkness of despair. Sometimes a tree
branch that is carrying more weight than it can bear will
become weak and gently lower itself onto a stronger branch
for support until it drops the weight onto the ground below.
Then it will lift itself up and grow stronger on its own. We
have an awesome responsibility today. Please do your part
today.

Prayer
God, help us be available to anybody who may need our
support today. Help us reach out to the person that may be
feeling suicidal so that they may hear the message of love,
recovery, and support. Amen

September 13

Thought for the day
If you are patient in one moment of anger, you will escape a hundred days of sorrow.

Chinese proverb

Meditation
When we are depressed, we often feel restless and irritable. As a result, we can become quick to pass judgement and grow very impatient with the people in our lives. By recognizing this behavior as a symptom of clinical depression, we stand a much better chance of avoiding the ensuing sorrow that we will create if we act out on these feelings. Anger always precedes sadness in my life because anger initially feels better. But sometimes my behavior while I am in denial about how I really feel can cause me many harms. It is painful to hurt the ones that we love, and it can feel shameful to later make the necessary amends. Today it is important for me to recognize these symptoms and to practice patience and tolerance in the times that I feel like striking out at others.

Prayer
God, help me today to practice patience and tolerance in all my affairs. Help me to understand how my displaced anger will always come back to hurt me. Amen

September 14

Thought for the day
If I am not for myself, who will be for me? And if I am only
for myself, what am I? And if not now, when?

Hillel

Meditation
I know now that I suffer from a disease, not a moral failure
or a lack of appreciation. I also know that I am responsible
for treating my disease with whatever tools work for me –
medication, support groups, therapy. I have to be on my side
first and foremost, and ignore those who would try to make
me feel "less than" for having the disease of depression. I
will remember that the same people who belittle mental
illnesses would never think of belittling the diabetic or the
kidney patient on dialysis or the one who suffers from
glaucoma – yet chronic illness is chronic illness, no matter
what organ is affected. I know too that I have a
responsibility to carry the message, to help others like myself
find the sunshine again and lose the shame others have
placed on them. To have a disease is not one's fault – but to
not treat it is.

Prayer
God, help me to remember that I have only today, only now.
If I want to make the most of this precious gift of today, I
must treat my illness first. Help me to live today according
to your will, secure in the knowledge of your love for me.
Amen

September 15

Thought for the day
In extreme youth, in our most humiliating sorrow, we think we are all alone. When we are older we find that others have suffered too.

Suzanne Moarny

Meditation
I have found much comfort in discovering that I am not alone with any of my trials and tribulations today. No matter what my sorrow or pain may be, I have discovered that there is always somebody who has already successfully worked through a similar experience...somebody who is now willing to share their experience, strength, and hope with me. Common bounds are wrought through common perils. We who suffer from this illness are currently part of a group of people that numbers in the hundreds of millions. Some of our members, ignorantly believing that they are still all alone, will unknowingly let this illness run its course throughout their life, and they will die from it. Today we must maintain the understanding that depression is an illness, which can isolate and kill us. We must be willing to reach out to the community of recovering people and partake in the comradery and fellowship that we so rightfully deserve.

Prayer
God thank you for the camaraderie and fellowship which I have found within my circle of support. Help me continue to build upon and trust these relationships while remaining available to anybody new who reaches out for help. Amen

September 16

Thought for the day
All happiness depends on courage and work. I have had many periods of wretchedness, but with energy and above all with illusions, I pulled through them all.

Honore de Balzac

Meditation
Maintaining a daily reprieve from depression requires a varying degree of effort on my part. Most of the time, the only reminder I have that I suffer from this disease is when I am taking my medication. Other times, it takes everything I have to get through the day without hurting myself. Our happiness today is contingent on our courage and effort. Some of us have been afflicted so badly that on occasion, we have missed a month of work at one time. Our employers usually have no idea what our problem is or what they should do with us. We can become embarrassed and ashamed to show our faces back at the office. What is sad about this is that if we had been sick with a more conventional illness such as pneumonia, we probably would have received flowers and cards of support in our absence. That being said, we need to accept that we are truly courageous to be willing to go to any length to take care of ourselves. We need to understand that we can and will pull though each and every bout with depression if we remain willing to do what is needed.

Prayer
God, today I pray for the willingness that I will need to treat my depression one day at a time for the rest of my life. I must accept my limitations today and understand that I must take care of myself before I can be of any service to anybody else. Amen

September 17

Thought for the day
It is terribly amusing how many different climates of feeling one can go through in a day.

Anne Morrow Lindbergh

Meditation
It is quite amusing for me to consider how often my emotions have dragged me by my nose across the roller-coaster tracks of life. Up and down with sudden twists and turns, only to come to an abrupt stop at the end of the day...as I lay my dizzy head upon my pillow. In my recovery, I have been learning how to gain control over how I feel by recognizing that my attitude and outlook can be adjusted to modify how I am feeling at any given moment. More importantly, I am becoming comfortable enough to sit back and occasionally enjoy the ride of my life. The problem we have when we are in the black hole is that our normal range of emotions is limited to feelings associated with despair. When we are afflicted, we are robbed of the pleasant feelings that can serve as a counterbalance to our depression. We become mired in emotions of rage and shame while feeling overwhelmed, lonely, jealous, confused, guilty, suspicious, frustrated, sad, embarrassed and disgusted. These feelings, although part of a healthy person's life, can become detrimental to our health, even fatal if left unchecked for any length of time.

Prayer
God, please help me pay attention to my feelings today. Help me use them to get a better understanding of what is happening within me so that I may modify my attitude and outlook toward life accordingly. Amen

September 18

Thought for the day
And when you're in a Slump
You're not in for much fun.
Un-slumping yourself
Is not easily done.
Dr. Seuss <u>Oh, the Places You'll Go!</u>

Meditation
How many times have you become extremely frustrated with yourself because you couldn't seem to "snap out" of your sadness? I know that hundreds of times I have tried to convince myself that my life really was not that bad and that my depressed mood just didn't make any sense. Today I know my despair was not the result of a poor attitude but rather a symptom of an illness. After years of treating this illness, I still find relief in knowing that I was not the rotten, ungrateful bastard I had made myself out to be. Yet knowing what was wrong was only half the battle. I still had to do the work that was required of me to un-slump myself, and as the verse indicates, it was not fun or easily done. Today we must remain willing to do what must be done if we find ourselves in another slump of depression.

Prayer
God, help me to remember that un-slumping myself will not always be easily done. Help me remember that I don't have to try to do it alone...that it is ok to call for help. Amen

September 19

Thought for the day
To affect the quality of the day - that is the highest of the arts.

Henry David Thoreau

Meditation
Today I treat my depression, not to prolong my eventual death, but to improve the quality of my life. I suffered for so long with days of despair...days that I was certain I was going to end it all. If I hope to continue to improve upon the quality of this day, then I must remain honest, open-minded, and willing to practice the high art of recovery. By taking care of myself, I allow myself the opportunity to reap the greatest reward that this life has to offer...the ability to affect the quality of another person's day.

Prayer
God, help me to be useful in another person's life today. Help me be a friend to anybody that needs somebody to lean on. Amen

September 20

Thought for the day
Muddy water, let stand, becomes clear.

Lao-tzu

Meditation
Sometimes all we need to do is STOP and be STILL. Instead of wallowing in our madness, we need to shut down the insane messages that the "village idiot" keeps posting on the information board between our ears, and in quiet prayer ask our Creator for guidance and inspiration as to what our next right move should be. I am quite capable of whipping myself into a mental frenzy of worry and despair over the simplest of daily chores. My wheels can spin so fast, that all I ever accomplish is digging myself into a deeper hole while kicking mud up on everything that surrounds me. Today when I find myself in the midst of my own clamor and confusion, I have to reluctantly confess that I am a mess and in desperate need of divine wisdom and understanding. Amazingly, if I turn to prayer and wait quietly for guidance, I soon intuitively know how to handle the problem that I once found so baffling.

Prayer
God, help me today to turn to you for guidance and inspiration before I make a mess out of something. Amen

September 21

Thought for the day
The greatest pleasure I know is to do a good action by
stealth, and to have it found out by accident.

Charles Lamb

Meditation
A key ingredient of my recovery today is my willingness to
be available to others who are suffering from this disease. I
have made it a practice to participate in a variety of support
groups within my community. Often I will meet a
"newcomer" who is standing on very unstable ground. They
may share how depressed they feel or discuss how they were
recently considering suicide. It is important to my recovery
that I make every effort to talk to this person about
depression and share with them my own experience,
strength, and hope. I need to give them my phone number
and encourage them to call me no matter how they are
feeling, but especially if they are feeling suicidal. I have
found that being a friend to others, whether they were
looking for one or not, has helped me to develop some really
great friendships. It is also important for me not to discuss
how I may be helping somebody out. First, it is nobody
else's business what problems the individual may be
experiencing. Second, it is important that I don't develop a
big fat head!

Prayer
God, help me today be available and helpful to others. Help
me to keep my ears open and listening for warning signs of
this disease. If I hear somebody talking about feelings of
worthlessness, grant me the courage to make myself
available in their lives. Amen

September 22

Thought for the day
"We cannot tell what may happen to us in the strange medley
of life. But we can decide what happens in us – how we take
it, what we do with it – and that is what really counts in the
end".

Joseph Fort Newton

Meditation
Today we are empowered to change how we take life – how
we handle it. We no longer have to react to every feeling
and emotion that creeps unexpectedly upon us. We have
gained new information that allows us the freedom to choose
whether or not we are going to react or act toward life's
peculiar twist and turns. What a liberating feeling I get when
I am able to stop myself from reacting to a situation with my
old behaviors and consider the alternative perspectives with
which I may now view my life.

Prayer
God thank you for the new perspectives I have gained as a
result of my recovery process. Thank you for the knowledge
that I now have regarding the illness of clinical depression.
Amen

September 23

Thought for the day
By yielding you may obtain victory.

Ovid

Meditation
For many of us, the idea of treating clinical depression is, for whatever reason, troublesome. For those of us who suffer from other addictions, the concern is usually centered around becoming "hooked" on the medication. We are worried that we may experience mood-altering reactions to the anti-depressant, reactions that may lead us back to our drug of choice. For others, the idea of taking any prescription medication for an extended period of time carries with it a stigma of weakness. It is amazing to me how quickly we are able to forget the suffering that we have been experiencing, when we come face to face with a proven solution to our dilemma. The first step toward relief from depression is to fully concede to our innermost self that we are afflicted. By acceptance, we may begin to obtain victory over this disease.

Prayer
God, please help me today to take care of myself in a healthy manner. Help me to recognize my fears of the unknown so that I may work through them toward a successful recovery from this disease. Amen

September 24

Thought for the day
What a lovely surprise to discover how un-lonely being alone can be.

Ellen Burstyn

Meditation
I had felt all alone for so many years. I recall many attempts to relieve myself of these depressed feelings of loneliness by trying to become involved with life. Whenever I would successfully infringe upon a circle of people in which I presumed I would gain feelings of acceptance and purpose, I would continue to harbor thoughts of phoniness and feelings of inferiority. Today I have grown to recognize that much of my purpose and character has been adversely affected by my untreated depression. I have since found that my need to "fit in" has proportionally decreased with each step I have taken toward uncovering my authentic self. By being restored to sane thinking, I no longer have to live with the lonely lies of phoniness and inadequacy that I now associate with being depressed.

Prayer
God, thank you for the progress I have made…progress that has freed me from the relentless press of feeling phony and alone. Thank you for all the people you have placed in my life…people that have encouraged me to reevaluate myself in a more healthy and positive way. Amen

September 25

Thought for the day
What a foe may do to a foe
Or a hater to a hater
Far worse that
The mind ill held may do to him
Chapter 3 The Mind, <u>Dhammapada</u>

Meditation
When we are suffering from any mental disorder, we can consider our mind as "ill". Left untreated, any mental illness will eventually harm our physical well-being. Clinical depression is no different in this matter. Many of us, unaware that we were suffering from a treatable illness, have attempted to take our own lives in a variety of ways. Whether it be a blatant suicide attempt or a more passive form of self-destruction, our ill mind becomes our greatest foe and supporter of self-hatred. Today we have learned to look upon our persistent pessimism and sadness as symptomatic of an ill mind that must be treated to prevent any future physical harm. We understand that it is appropriate to seek medical attention for our ailment as readily as we would for a physical concern.

Prayer
God, please help all who are suffering from this illness to seek the medical attention they need to relieve themselves of their "ill" mind. Help them to recognize that it is appropriate to treat a mental medical condition as readily as they would a physical one. Amen

September 26

Thought for the day
Every now and again take a good look at something not made with hands – a mountain, a star, the turn of a stream. There will come to you wisdom and patience and solace and, above all, the assurance that you are not alone in the world.

Sidney Lovett

Meditation
Today it is very important that we become willing to dispute the loneliness produced by clinical depression with the reality that we are not alone in the world. There is much to be said for the positive impact taking in the awesome splendor of nature can have on our outlook toward life. It is important to my recovery that I occasionally partake in a leisurely stroll through the woods or enjoy peaceful wonderment as I gaze into the star filled skies of the night. We need to continually practice new methods of improving our spiritual condition so that the lies of depression no longer coincide with our new way of thinking about ourselves and the world in which we presently live.

Prayer
God, help me make the time I need today to stop and smell the roses in my life. Help me realize that by creating the time I need for myself, I become well suited to be helpful to others. Amen

September 27

Thought for the day
If you work on your mind with your mind, how can you
avoid an immense confusion?

Seng–ts an

Meditation
Many of us have wasted numerous years of our lives and
countless amounts of energy trying to self-diagnose and then
"fix" ourselves.   In the process, we lost out on many
opportunities to enjoy our life, and perhaps even destroyed
parts of it that we held dear to our hearts. We added to the
confusion that was already prevalent in our minds by
creating more chaos while we were busy pointing our fingers
at everything we presumed was causing our persistent
sadness. The question of "if you work on your mind with
your mind, how can you avoid an immense confusion", is a
fair question to ask. If my way of thinking is distorted by an
untreated mental illness, then it is correct for me to assume
that until I receive treatment for that illness, my thinking will
remain distorted.   The confusion that surrounded my
depression began to disperse the moment I accepted medical
attention and began to treat it as I would any other illness.

Prayer
God, for many of us, it has been difficult to accept our
depression as a treatable medical condition rather than a poor
attitude that we have to change on our own. There are still
those, even within the medical community, that consider the
use of anti-depressant medications as nothing more than a
mask and a way to cover up the "real" problem. Help all of
us who are involved with this illness, no matter in what
capacity, to continue in our efforts to learn and understand
all that there is to know about this potentially fatal, yet
treatable condition. Amen

September 28

Thought for the day
I now choose to rise above my personality problems to recognize the magnificence of my being. I am totally willing to learn to love myself.

Louise L. Hay

Meditation
Did clinical depression contribute to my personality problems? You bet it did! Depression deprived me of self-love, without which I became a very insecure, unloving person. Even when people in my life would go to extraordinary lengths to shower me with affection, I would quickly discount their words of encouragement and signs of love as unmerited and therefore not authentic. Today, by execution of our choice to recognize that we are all truly magnificent beings, we have begun the process of learning how to love ourselves.

Prayer
God, help me today to rise above all obstacles that may stand in my way of overcoming my personality problems. Help me recognize that I am a magnificent being who deserves to continue to learn how to love others and himself. Amen

September 29

Thought for the day
I am not afraid of storms for I am learning how to sail my ship.

Louisa May Alcott

Meditation
My life can become extremely stormy if I allow my past poisonous pedagogy to guide the way. Whether self-taught or inherited, the toxic teachings of yesterday have no business at the helm of my life today. I have been blessed with a new set of instruments and navigational instructions that will safely see me through the darkest of unrest by directing me to the serenity of a peaceful harbor. I have surrendered to the idea that my previous belief system will ever aim me in the direction of peaceful waters, but rather continually place me in dangerous seas.

Prayer
God thank you for the lessons I have learned which now allow me to sail on safe seas. Thank you for the courage to rid myself of my old belief systems and replace them with a new set of navigational instructions. Amen

September 30

Thought for the day
Great Spirit, help me never to judge another until I have walked in his moccasins.

Sioux Indian Prayer

Meditation
We have all been critical of somebody else at one time or another. We certainly have been critical of ourselves...and others also have judged us, perhaps unfairly. Many of us, while suffering from a bout with depression, have become victims of judgement and sometimes condemnation from the people that we work or live with. From their vantage point, we appear ungrateful and perhaps pitifully childish because of our seeming unwillingness to "pull ourselves together". We often have become extremely angry at their inability to show compassion and understanding toward our condition. In both instances, the tension could be subdued if only both parties would try to walk in each other's moccasins for awhile. Today, I no longer have the time or energy to spend trying to convince others to understand me. It is better for me to be content to just walk in their moccasins for a bit. By doing so, I can understand how and why they don't understand me, and by recognizing this, I may know peace.

Prayer
Great Spirit, help me never to judge another until I have walked in his moccasins. Amen

October 1

Thought for the day
Be not afraid of growing slowly,
Be afraid only of standing still.
Chinese proverb

Meditation
I have discovered that I tend to make my personal growth in spurts rather than experiencing slow continuous progression. When my pain becomes great, I will seek out the help I need. Once I begin to make another journey of self-exploration, I often end up going deeper into myself than I had initially planned. I frequently come out of my journey with a new set of beliefs by which I may live my life. I am usually very excited about the progress that I have made, and I am always eager to share my experiences with others. But often, after the newness has worn off, I find myself becoming complacent. I believe it is acceptable for me to enjoy the fruits of my effort for a little while, but it is very important that I do not rest on my laurels for long. I have learned that my spiritual growth is a process, not an event. Therefore I must remain willing to continue to grow slowly, and maintain a healthy fear of standing still for any great length of time.

Prayer
God, help me today to take action to maintain my spiritual growth. Help me to not grow complacent and rest on my laurels. Amen

October 2

Thought for the day
We cannot climb up a rope that is attached only to our own belt.

William Ernest Hocking

Meditation
I can imagine myself standing in a gymnasium with one end of a rope attached to my belt loop and the remaining length coiled up in my hand, repeatedly heaving the rope upward in an attempt to lasso a hook that is hanging off the rafter twenty feet above. I first determine that the problem is there is not enough weight at the end of the rope to propel it to the height of the hook. So I busily search and find a small weight that I rapidly tape onto the end of the rope. As I resume my attempt to lasso the hook, I find that my rope now has the weight needed to repeatedly hit the hook, but by doing so, I discover the hook is not stationary therefore giving way each time the rope hits it. I realize that I must produce a perfect toss if I ever hope to secure my rope onto the hook above. As I continue with my attempts, my neck grows tired from my constant upward stare. Also, I notice that the two maintenance men who have been diligently replacing all the light bulbs in the gym are moving very close to the area where I am standing. Concerned about my falling rope hitting one of the men on the head, I agree to take a break until they are finished. It never dawns on me to ask the man with the ladder to hook the rope for me! How important is it for us to learn how to ask for help today?

Prayer
God, please grant me the courage to ask for help when I need it. Help me remember that I don't have to accomplish every task on my own...that it is not a sign of weakness, but rather a sign of wisdom to ask for help. Amen

October 3

Thought for the day
Your vision will become clear only when you can look into your own heart.

Carl Jung

Meditation
When I was still undiagnosed, there was a conflict waging between my heart and my mind. The latter repeatedly told me I was worthless and deserved to die, and the former said that God loved me and would continue to love me whether I loved myself or not. Seemingly unable to bring the two into accord, I felt as though I were truly going insane. Today I accept that when I am suffering from depression my thinking is less than what the psychiatric community would consider sane. Understanding that depression indicates my mind is ill allows me the opportunity to take appropriate steps to restore myself to sane thinking.

Prayer
God, help me today to lead with my heart and not with my mind. Amen

October 4

Thought for the day
The past has flown away. The coming month and year do not exist. Ours only is the present's tiny point.

Mahmud Shabistari

Meditation
Our life today is an accumulation of our present tiny points. By beginning to improve the condition of our present, we create for ourselves a much more attractive past to reflect upon. Treating our depression is key to our ability to successfully improve our present condition. We can't expect to experience days of healing if we are doing nothing to bring about such changes in our life. It is best for us today to let "worry" worry about worry, and let the past tend to the past, while we work toward living in this moment.

Prayer
God, please help me let go of the past and free me from the worry of tomorrow so that I may rejoice in this moment with which you have blessed me. Amen

October 5

Thought for the day
If we do not change our direction, we are likely to end up
where we are headed.

Chinese proverb

Meditation
In what direction are you headed today? Are you slipping
into a period of depression and ignoring all the warning
signs? Are you hoping to pull yourself out of your funk? Do
you plan to suffer through another day in the hopes that you
will feel a little better tomorrow? Have you been avoiding
your friends by turning down offers to socialize? It is
important for all of us to remember that a bout with
depression usually does not hit us like a ton of bricks...it
creeps upon us without our knowledge. Slowly we slip
toward the black hole and then WHAM! We are lost again.
Today we must pay attention to the direction in which we are
heading. If you recognize the symptoms, get the help you
need immediately. I believe that you probably have suffered
enough already.

Prayer
God, please help us all to recognize and take the appropriate
action as soon as we notice the symptoms of depression in
our lives. Amen

October 6

Thought for the day
We should have much peace if we would not busy ourselves
with the sayings and doings of others.

Thomas a Kempis

Meditation
It is very easy to lose our focus on ourselves and become
busy with what others are doing and saying. Many people
spend their entire lives pointing out what is wrong with
everybody else without ever taking the time to consider that
they too play a role in all that is happening in their life. I
know such people, and frankly, I can't stand to be around
them much any more. It's not personal, I just find that the
most interesting people today are the people who spend their
time focusing on changing themselves rather than avoiding
themselves by pointing fingers at others. We know that prior
to being diagnosed with clinical depression, many of us,
myself included, spent way too much time pointing fingers
and blaming others for our sad state rather than taking
responsibility for ourselves and seeking treatment. Today,
before I accuse you of anything, I know that I need to first
take a look at myself.

Prayer
God, it can be so easy to backslide into a life of self-
avoidance by becoming a busybody know-it-all. Help me
today to avoid that very unattractive trap. Help me to worry
about myself and leave the rest of the world in your more-
than-capable hands. Amen

299

October 7

Thought for the day
The ability to simplify means to eliminate the unnecessary so that the necessary may speak.

Hans Hofmann

Meditation
Over the years, many of us have accumulated the excess "baggage" that is frequently associated with untreated clinical depression. By believing the lies of this illness for so long, we lived a life that was a magnet for "garbage thinking". Feelings of worthlessness begot feelings of worthlessness, and so we continually added false evidence onto our wagon of hopelessness and despair. It is not easy to rid ourselves of our unnecessary low self-esteem and replace it with a necessary healthy self-image, but if we are now treating this illness, we too have the ability to simplify our lives by no longer perpetuating the lies of this disease.

Prayer
God, help me today to simplify my life by eliminating the unnecessary "baggage" that I have been carrying with me for so long. Help me to know a life that consists of enjoying that which is necessary by leaving the unnecessary alone. Amen

October 8

Thought for the day
We are what we repeatedly do. Excellence, then, is not an act, but a habit.

Aristotle

Meditation
If I repeatedly reach out for help when I feel myself slipping into a period of depression, then it can be said that I am a person who possesses self-love and cares about his well being. If I repeatedly try to help others that are afflicted with this illness, then it can be said that I am a helpful person. If I repeatedly turn to my Creator for guidance and inspiration, then it can be said that I am a faithful believer in the divine wisdom of my God.

Prayer
God, help me today to repeatedly do those things which will lead me toward spiritual excellence in my life. Amen

October 9

Thought for the day
My imperfections and failures are as much a blessing from God as my successes and my talents, and I lay them both at His feet.

Mahatma Gandhi

Meditation
I can say with complete certainty that if it were not for my imperfections and failures, I would not be as concerned with my spiritual condition as I am today. It was by being brought to my knees by the insanity of depression, that I turned to God in prayer. There I began a spiritual journey that has left me in awe of God's everlasting love and merciful saving grace. I since have learned to expect God to continue to work miracles in my life by working through the people He has placed into my life to help me continue to find my way along this road of happy destiny.

Prayer
God, I stand before you today just as I am. I ask you to help me overcome my imperfections and failures so that I may become more useful to you. Amen

October 10

Thought for the day
The ultimate lesson all of us have to learn is unconditional love, which includes not only others but ourselves as well.

Elizabeth Kubler-Ross

Meditation
Perhaps the most difficult wound that our depression has left us to heal, is the wound of self-hatred. It has cut deep within the fabric of our existence leaving behind a severely damaged self-esteem. Left unchecked, our self-hatred eventually permeated into every relationship we had, but especially our relationship with ourselves. Upon beginning our recovery, we soon discover that we know very little about unconditional love and self-love. By accepting that we do not feel love for ourselves, we allow ourselves the opportunity to become open-minded and willing to take direction...direction that will help us to begin to heal. If we are willing to practice a new way of thinking about ourselves, one day at a time, we will slowly learn to love ourselves. Once we learn self-love we can begin to learn life's ultimate lesson...the lesson of how to love unconditionally.

Prayer
God, please help all of us who struggle to repair our self-esteem. Help us to practice new ways to think about ourselves so that we may know self-love. Amen

October 11

Thought for the day
When we long for life without...difficulties, remind us that
oaks grow strong in contrary winds and diamonds are made
under pressure.

Peter Marshall

Meditation
Am I a better person today than I would have been had I not
endured all the adversity that has been in my life? I believe
that I am. But does that mean I should welcome my trials
and tribulations as opportunities for personal growth? When
my spiritual condition is fit and my faith strong, I would
answer yes. But it is not often that I find myself in that
space, so new obstacles in my life are usually initially met
with feelings of disappointment and frustration. It is easy for
me to convince myself that, because of the efforts I have
made to reclaim my life I should somehow be shielded from
all future problems. When I find myself longing for a life
that is free from difficulties, I must remember that life does
not stand still for me. If I find myself in a comfortable spot,
I should try to enjoy it as long as it lasts...but I must
understand that it will not last forever. Life goes on...and
with its motion, problems do arise. The best I can strive for
today is to learn how to live life on life's term's one day at a
time.

Prayer
God, help me understand that many of my problems today
are opportunities for spiritual growth. Help me to take
advantage of these opportunities so that I may continue to
improve upon my character. Amen

October 12

Thought for the day
Always remember that no matter what the problem may be, there is an infinity of solutions.

Marion Weinstein

Meditation
The good news we share with each other today is that we no longer have to suffer from depression. Treatment is available...if we realize we are depressed. That is where the problem still lies for most of us. Even though we have been diagnosed with this illness and have received treatment for it in the past, it is common for us, upon feeling better, to think that we are now "cured". It is important that we accept that we might experience reoccurring episodes of depression throughout the rest of our lives. We need to familiarize ourselves with all the possible symptoms that depression can exhibit, and be willing to take the appropriate action if we discover any of these symptoms becoming prevalent in our lives.

Prayer
God, help me remember that if the problems associated with depression begin to creep back into my life...there is an infinity of solutions available to me if I am being honest with myself regarding how I am actually feeling. Amen

October 13

Thought for the day
Nothing is troublesome that we do willingly.

Thomas Jefferson

Meditation
My willingness to accept myself as I am is the master key in which I may continually use to unlock the doors of self-awareness in my life. My willingness to change the things I find disturbing about myself allows me to continue growing spiritually in my recovery. There was a time in my life when everything I did felt like a burden. Everything felt troublesome, even receiving treatment for my depression, because I had very little willingness left inside me. Most of it had been left within the wreckage of my past. Ironically, my depression sapped me of my willingness, the very thing I needed to treat my depression. Acceptance has turned out to be that which will replenish me of willingness whenever I am running low. By accepting clinical depression as a disease, I was able to muster enough willingness to begin to treat it.

Prayer
God, please help me today to maintain the willingness that I need to do those things which need to be done...whether I want to do them or not. Amen

October 14

Thought for the day
It is wealth to be content.
Lao-tsu

Meditation
Peace of mind, a sense of security and well being,
contentment...these are the fruits that have led me...season
after season...to cultivate the soils of my mind, heart and
soul. As long as the yield exceeds the effort, I will continue
to work my land. Faith tells me that all my tears were not in
vain...that they prepared the way in which I now grow.

Prayer
God thank you for the realization I now have that my toil and
sweat was not a worthless effort...that today, I can bring
forth goodness out of my painful past. Amen

October 15

Thought for the day
Listen to your feelings. They tell you when you need to take care of yourself, like finding a friend if you feel lonely, crying if you feel sad, singing and smiling if you feel happy, and acting frisky if you feel good.

Pat Palmer

Meditation
Today, make a conscious decision to become aware of the range of feelings that you experience throughout your day. Write them down on a piece of paper. In the evening, before you go to bed, refer to your list. Were you sad, glad, mad, or fearful today? Did one particular emotion dominate over the others? Practice this exercise daily for one week. At the end of the week, review your accumulated information. Do you notice a trend of any type? Do certain circumstances always bring out the same emotions in you or do you find that you can react quite differently to similar events from day to day? If feelings of sadness, worthlessness, despair, pessimism, and even anger headline your list, then you may be suffering from depression without realizing it. It is very important that I practice listening to my feelings each day. By practicing over the past few years, I now have the ability to quickly understand when I am experiencing the symptoms of depression, and can more readily do something about it.

Prayer
God, help me today to practice listening to my feelings. Help me work through the "fronts" that I often use to deny my true emotions...fronts that hide me from the truth about what is really going on inside of me. Amen

October 16

Thought for the day
Planning is deciding what to change today so tomorrow will
be different from yesterday.

Ichak Adizes

Meditation
When I identify a pattern of thought or behavior that I find
detrimental to my mental and physical health, it is important
that I set about to determine a course of action, which will
relieve me of what I now find unacceptable. Coming up
with a realistic plan to change can sometimes become more
challenging then the change itself. Often times, I will set
myself up with an elaborate scheme of bells and whistles that
I could not possibly manage on my own. When my plan
then fails, I conclude that I tried to change, but just couldn't
do it. Today I must be certain that I possess the character
traits that will be required to produce the changes in my life
that I desire. One of the fastest ways for me to take
inventory of my character is with a close friend in recovery
or a therapist. By discussing what I think I need to change in
my life to improve it, and sharing my plan of action with
another person, I become open to suggestions that may save
me a lot of time and even pain.

Prayer
God, help me continue to discover the things in my life that I
need to change. Help me use the support I now have to
devise and implement a plan of action that will bring forth
the desired results. Amen

October 17

Thought for the day
The time you enjoy wasting is not wasted time.

Bertrand Russell

Meditation
After considering today's thought for a few moments, I realized that I frequently equate playful time as wasteful time. I sometimes find it very difficult to relax and just do things for the sheer purpose of enjoyment. I can become so entwined in my pursuit of the deeper meanings of life that I miss out on the many opportunities I have to just kick up my heels and laugh awhile. It is important for me today to make some recreational time for myself. I need to have a time where I can just relax and have some fun. Of course when I am depressed, the desire to actually have fun is almost non-existent, so it is important that I take care of first things first. But I can say that in the past, I have found a little comic relief can do wonders for my spirit.

Prayer
God, help me today to make the time to have some fun. Help me learn how to relax and not take every moment of my life so seriously. Amen

October 18

Thought for the day
God seems to have the receiver off the hook.

Arthur Koestler

Meditation
There have been many times in my life when I have completely given up on God. I used to pour my heart out in desperate prayer...begging for forgiveness and mercy...asking him to relieve me of the bondage of self. Hoping that he would miraculously appear in my life, causing a revolutionary upheaval that would somehow transform me from the wretched sinner that I was, into a saint. After finishing my prayer, I would sit and wait for some imaginary feeling to consume me...and when it didn't, I would slip deeper into my despair because I had no where else to go. Today I have the faith that all my prayers have been and will continue to be answered, but they are answered on God's time...in God's way. More importantly, I have come to understand that sometimes God's answer is No. I must accept that answer today with the faith that God's plan for me is far superior to any plan I may have contrived on my own.

Prayer
God, help me today to see how miraculously you are working in my life even when I do not "feel" your presence. Help me accept that when you answer my prayers with a "No" it is because your knowledge of what is best for me is superior to any plan I may contrive on my own. Amen

October 19

Thought for the day
Give God time.
                    The Koran

Meditation
For years I have listened to people who have preceded me
along this path of recovery, say that I should not quit before
the miracle happens. Initially, I felt as though these people
were perhaps a bit smitten with illusions of white rabbits,
candy houses and angels hovering about them every step of
their way. I expected that my life might improve, but I was
no longer anticipating that I might be blinded by my
Creator's awesome light. As I look back, I can see how,
once again, my perceptions of reality and my expectations
were distorted. God has worked miracles in my life. But
these miracles have occurred slowly, as many miracles in life
do. If I compare where I am at today to yesterday, I don't
really see much difference. But when I compare myself
today to four years ago, then I can say there is truly a loving
God who has worked miraculously in my life. The fact that I
did not die from clinical depression, but turned to treatment,
not 100% willingly I might add, is evidence enough for me
today that there is a Great Spirit working in our lives.

Prayer
God, please help me to be patient and trusting of your divine
wisdom and power today. Help me understand what actions
I need to take to successfully carry out your will for my life.
Amen

October 20

Thought for the day
The meaning of good and bad, of better and worse, is simply helping or hurting.

Ralph Waldo Emerson

Meditation
A good tool we can use to help us "self-check" where we are in our recovery process, is to periodically stop and ask ourselves whether what we are doing or what we are planning to do, is helping or hurting us. It is important for me to also include another person in this form of self-appraisal because, often times, I can be hurting myself with nothing but the best intentions without even realizing it. The same holds true when I am helping others. As the saying goes, the road to hell is paved with good intentions. I have to always be honest with myself regarding my motives for helping somebody else. If I discover, or if somebody points out to me, that my intentions appear to be less than pure, then I should back off because if I continue, not only will I be hurting another person, but I will also be hurting myself.

Prayer
God, help me today to pay attention to whether I am helping or hurting myself. If I find myself sabotaging my life, grant me the courage to call for help before I continue down a path of depression and self-destruction. When I am helping others, help me to continually evaluate whether my motives are pure or not. If I find that they are less then honorable, help me to back away from the situation as quickly as possible so that two people don't end up hurt. Amen

October 21

Thought for the day
So often we search out the impossible-and then throw
ourselves into trying to do it.

Anonymous

Meditation
The agony and despair I went through when I was suffering
from clinical depression without being aware that I was
afflicted with the disease nearly ended my life on more than
one occasion. I tried so hard to change...I hated myself for
being such a failure, but no matter what I did to make things
better in my life, I always seemed to end up back in the same
sad, pitiful state of mind. I didn't realize it at the time, but I
was trying to accomplish the impossible. I was trying to
make myself happy again by improving (or changing) my
surroundings. I was trying to accomplish and achieve things
that would prove my self-worth. It seemed that the harder I
tried, the harder I fell. Over the years, my willingness to try
to lift out of my sadness weakened substantially, and
consequently I got to the point were I just stayed down. As a
depression sufferer, I have to be aware of when I might be
setting myself up to fail. I have to pay attention to how
much hope I am placing in a person or event to make me feel
happy.

Prayer
God, help me to avoid setting myself up for failure. Help me
recognize that when I am depressed, the remedy will come
from within me. Amen

October 22

Thought for the day
Have patience with all things, but first of all with yourself.

Francis de Sales

Meditation
Our depression has caused us to be so hard on ourselves for so long. We have become accustomed to living our lives with such disparagement that it is sometimes difficult for us to give ourselves a break. Even though we are now treating this illness and our bottom has raised up a bit, we still can find it very difficult to treat ourselves with dignity and respect. To be patient with myself means I must first care about myself. When I get stuck in my old way of thinking, I have to remind myself that I didn't cause this disease. It is not my fault that I suffer from it. I did not do something bad that somehow contributed to my becoming afflicted. I also have to remember that I do not have to convince anybody of the authenticity of how I feel when I am depressed. Today, all I have to do is walk beside my brothers and sisters who suffer from this illness, and share whatever it is of me that may be of some use to them.

Prayer
God, help me today to be patient and tolerant of myself. Help me remember that it is not my fault that I am afflicted with this disease and that I do not have to convince anyone of its authenticity. Amen

October 23

Thought for the day
You are a child of the universe, no less than the trees and the
stars; you have a right to be here. And whether or not it is
clear to you, no doubt the universe is unfolding as it should.

Max Ehrmann

Meditation
When I am trapped by depression, the idea that I have a right
to be in the world of light and peace is laughable. I only feel
like I am entitled to die. But that is my disease telling its
black lies to me. "What is the point?" I cry. The point is
that I am here either to teach a lesson or learn a lesson, and
even in the depths, there are lessons to be shared. What they
may be I don't always know, but there is a purpose to every
moment and breath. Knowing that I am gifted with a
purpose makes me a true child of the universe. I do have a
right to be here and a right to be happy. With a little faith
and a little work, I can once again look up at the trees and the
stars.

Prayer
God, help me to learn my lessons and to share my
experiences with other sufferers. Let me find my purpose
there. Amen

October 24

Thought for the day
Once you say you're going to settle for second, that's what happens to you in life, I find.

John F. Kennedy

Meditation
When I am convinced that I do not deserve to win the race...to finish first, then the best I can ever hope for is second place. When I am depressed, I rapidly become depleted of all self-confidence to succeed in life. I also fall into the trap of "all or nothing" thinking, where if I don't finish first, then I finish last. It is an important part of my recovery today to be on the lookout for this sort of mindset because it is a recipe for disaster. I must continually practice believing that I do not have to settle for second best in my life any more. But if my best efforts to succeed only yield me a second place finish, then I need to be proud of that accomplishment. Our untreated depression has spent years carving into thoughts the belief that we were good-for-nothing losers. We cannot expect to completely change this thinking overnight, but we can begin to erase this lie by getting honest with ourselves about all of our strengths and weaknesses, and then setting about achieving our own victories in life.

Prayer
God, my "all or nothing" thinking has caused me much grief in my life. Help me today to understand that my life is not to be rigid and unforgiving...that if I do my best and believe in myself, then I can find happiness in all that I accomplish regardless of what place I finish. Amen

October 25

Thought for the day
To be happy, we must not be too concerned with others.

Albert Camus

Meditation
When I am feeling bad, it is so easy for me to obsess on what other people are doing or saying...especially what they might be saying about me. I can recall many times in my life when I completely lost touch with myself because I was so busy trying to find out who other people thought I was. When we are trying to be "people pleasers" to gain our self-worth, we are stamping "welcome" across our backs and becoming a doormat for the world to wipe its feet on. Today I must not concern myself so much with what other people may be doing and saying, and just keep the focus on myself. Once I do this, I begin to realize that most people don't really find my life all that intriguing because, just like me, they have problems of their own.

Prayer
God, help me today to keep my focus inward. Help me treat my depression with all the proven methods that you have made available to me, rather than looking toward other people in my life to validate me and make me feel better. Amen

October 26

Thought for the day
Hate is consequence of fear; we fear something before we hate it; a child who fears noises becomes a man who hates noise.

Cyril Connolly

Meditation
Prior to accepting my condition and following the direction of others, I lived in fear. It has taken a few years for me to fully understand this, but upon a thorough investigation of my character, I have discovered that fear has been at the root of most of my disenchanting emotions. Consequently, I was a very hateful, vengeful human being. What I didn't understand at the time, but what I know today, is that all that hate I felt toward the outside world was really an expression of my hate for me. The first step of my recovery, which has turned out to be a daily, ongoing exercise, is to rid myself of the hate and concentrate on relieving myself of my root fears. Faith in God and the treatment that I have received have turned out to be my greatest resources to accomplish this on a daily basis. When I examine my thinking while I am depressed, I can see that fear of life is the driving force behind my thoughts of self-destruction. Today, I must be willing to talk about my fears with my friends in the recovering community and, if necessary, my doctor. By doing so, I am able to find the support and comfort that I need to overcome my fears and free myself of the hate that I was once so accustomed with.

Prayer
God, help me today to live free from the fears that have masqueraded as hate for so many years in my life. Amen

October 27

Thought for the day
History is a vast early warning system.

Norman Cousins

Meditation
For many of us, our history is not one that we are very proud
of...yet it can offer us great help today. Often, I use my past
as an example of how I don't want to live my life. I'm no
longer willing to waste any more time repeating the same
mistakes over and over again, expecting different results.
While I may not have all the answers to the riddles of my
life, my history frequently tells me what is not the right
answer...so that I may focus my attention on discovering
what the correct solution is for my life. It is insane thinking
if I believe that "this time it will be different" and proceed to
repeat an action that has proven harmful in my past...yet
many of us have done just that when it comes to dealing with
our depression. We have repeatedly tried to "will" ourselves
into feeling better, whether by trying to ignore our problem
or by manipulating others. Today I understand that my
history can be one of my greatest resources if I understand
that it should be used as a vast early warning system and not
a way of life.

Prayer
God, help me today to use my past in a matter that will be
beneficial to my recovery. Help me learn from my mistakes
and understand that if I do the same thing over and over
again...it would be foolish for me to expect different results.
Amen

October 28

Thought for the day
An act of God was defined as something which no
reasonable man could have expected.

A.P. Herbert

Meditation
I was absolutely convinced that I was to die from my
cocktail of depression, alcoholism, and cocaine addiction. I
was certain that God had abandoned me and that there was
no hope of ever drawing a sober breath again. Every time I
would try to stop drinking and using cocaine, I would slip
into such a deep, suicidal state of mind, that the only thing I
knew how to do to relieve my pain and suffering was to
drink and 'use'...which in time, only led to more pain and
suffering. If you had told me five years ago that I would still
be alive today doing the things that I am doing, I would have
laughed right in your face as I poured another drink down
my throat. I could not have planned how things have turned
out in my life, and I certainly had no reason left to expect a
resuscitation of my spirit...yet here I am, truly by the grace
of God, alive and sober, treating depression, one day at a
time.

Prayer
God thank you for the resuscitation of my spirit. Please
breathe hope into the spirits of all my brothers and sisters
who are still struggling to believe that they will ever know a
better life. Amen

October 29

Thought for the day
Everyone who has ever built anywhere a "new heaven" first
found the power thereto in his own hell.

Friedrich Nietzsche

Meditation
We all are familiar with our own hell. Some of us have lived
in it for so long that we have become comfortable in its
familiarity. But as we begin to recover from years of
personal neglect, we find that living in our own hell is no
longer acceptable to us. We find ourselves yearning for
relief from our depressed outlook on life...wanting only to
know a "new heaven" on which we may begin to build upon.
Recovery is about turning our pain into power. I was
powerless prior to being diagnosed with clinical depression.
After fighting the doctor's opinion for some time, I finally
surrendered to the fact that he may be correct in his
assessment of what was ailing me. By accepting my
condition, I placed myself in the position to readily receive
treatment, and it has been within my treatment process that I
became empowered to leave my own hell behind and begin
to build my new life.

Prayer
God thank you for the empowerment that I have discovered
by accepting myself as I am. Thank you for the knowledge
that I no longer have to live in my own hell...that through
acceptance I can continue to build my life within a "new
heaven". Amen

October 30

Thought for the day
Science may have found a cure for most evils: but it has found no remedy for the worst of them all – the apathy of human beings.

Helen Keller

Meditation
We can add apathy to the long list of personality traits that are associated with the clinically depressed. When we are suffering, we become disinterested with our surroundings and unresponsive to our inner voice that is crying out for help. Having been beaten down by this illness so many times, we have learned not to get our hopes up any more. We feel defeated...as if we could not make a difference in life even if we tried, so we give up. Many of us have experienced an apathetic outlook. When we slip into a period of depression, it is very difficult for us to not fall into the realm of the spiritless. But, by the grace of God, today we have each other. If we continue to reach out to one another for comfort and support, we create a powerful antidote for apathy...love.

Prayer
God, help me today to guard myself from the spiritless life that apathetic thinking has to offer. Help all of us who are trying to recover from depression continue to reach out to each other for comfort and support. Amen

October 31

Thought for the day
The greatest right in the world is the right to be wrong.

Harry Weinberger

Meditation
I have lived with the fear of being wrong much of my life. I am no longer concerned with how this fear originated, but I am deeply interested in continuing the relief that I have experienced apart from this burden. I have recognized that when I am enjoying a high sense of self-esteem, my need to prove my point and convince another that I am right decreases in direct proportion to my degree of self-worth. Likewise, if my self-esteem is in the gutter, my need to be right increases. It is important for me today to recognize that when I feel an overwhelming need to be right or make another see things my way, I can consider the desire as evidence that my self-esteem is probably not where it should be at that moment. By understanding this, I can get off the debating committee and focus my efforts on taking care of myself.

Prayer
God, please help me remember that I do not have to be perfect today...that it is acceptable for me to make mistakes. Amen

November 1

Thought for the day
After the game, the king and pawn go into the same box.

Italian proverb

Meditation
It is estimated that twenty million people in this country suffer from depression...and of that twenty million, thirty thousand commit suicide each year. Depression is an equal opportunity destroyer that knows no age, gender, race, or religious boundary. Whether you come from Yale or jail...the Parkway or the park bench, depression may strike upon you without you even realizing it. It is important for us to remember that suffering from clinical depression is not a flaw in our character. We need to share that message with everybody we may be talking with about this illness. We need to remember that whether we are kings or pawns, or anything in between, when it comes to treating this disease, we're all together in the "same box".

Prayer
God, help me today to be available to anybody that may need my help and support. Help me carry the message of hope whenever the opportunity presents itself. Amen

November 2

Thought for the day
The human body experiences a powerful gravitational pull in the direction of hope. That is why the patient's hopes are the physician's secret weapon. They are the hidden ingredients in any prescription.

Norman Cousins

Meditation
We greatly enhance our rate of recovery each day by working toward changing our attitude to one of gratitude. Each day that we successfully practice refuting the lies of depression, and replace our negative self-talk with that of hopeful, positive thinking, we improve our chances of meeting our next bout with the confidence that we can work through it. By letting go of our old ideas, and allowing the shared experiences of others to become influential in our lives, we begin to be drawn by the gravitational pull of recovery and a new way of life.

Prayer
God, help me today to experience an attitude of gratitude. Help me remember that by successfully refuting the lies of depression on a daily basis, I stand a much better chance of working through my next bout with this disease. Amen

November 3

Thought for the day
Man's mind stretched to a new idea never goes back to its
original dimensions.

Oliver Wendell Holmes

Meditation
I can remember the day I was approached with the "new
idea" that I might be suffering from clinical depression. I
can remember my initial revolt against the prospect that I
might have to take medication to find some relief. I recall a
few hopeless days later when I realized that I really had
nothing left to lose…that I surely would be dead within a
week if I continued on my path of hell-bent self-destruction.
I remember sitting in church a few days later, becoming
overwhelmed with the idea that maybe, just maybe,
untreated depression was the missing piece to my
puzzle…that if I began to treat my depression I might
develop the willingness I seemed to be lacking to maintain
continuous sobriety. I began to treat my illness that day and,
by the grace of God, I haven't had a drink since. My mind
was stretched with a new idea, an idea that has, up to this
moment, saved my life.

Prayer
God, help me continue in my efforts to elevate my mind and
get myself together. Amen

November 4

Thought for the day
Of all our faults, the one that we excuse most easily is
idleness.

La Rochefoucauld

Meditation
It is so easy to fall into the trap of complacency and stand
idle while the symptoms of depression begin to unfold before
our very eyes. This illness, by its very nature, has the ability
to take away our motivation to do anything to counteract its
symptoms. As we allow ourselves to slip deeper into the
black hole, the challenge to help ourselves becomes more
and more difficult. The results of idleness, as it pertains to
clinical depression, can be deadly. We cannot just stand by
and allow this disease to run amuck in our lives any longer.
We must be determined to remain ever watchful for all the
warning signs, and be prepared to execute a plan of action as
soon as we notice that we are in the shadows again.

Prayer
God, help me today not to assume that I am cured from
depression. Help me remember that this illness may strike
upon me at any time...that I need to have a plan of action in
place to execute when I find myself in the shadows again.
Amen

November 5

Thought for the day
As long as you live, keep learning how to live.

Seneca

Meditation
I am often very anxious to "know it all" so that I may sit back, relax, and enjoy the rest of my life. Unfortunately, that is not how life works. I have to be in a state of continual growth because growth is the only evidence I have of life. Each new day brings forth the opportunity to improve upon myself physically, mentally, and spiritually. Just as a garden, I need to tend to my life on a daily basis. By doing so, it is then fair for me to expect a garden free from weeds and bountiful with a useful crop. If I choose to become lazy and complacent, then it would be unfair for me to expect anything but a life full of useless weeds. The weeds can have one benefit to my life if I open my mind to it. They can serve as a reminder that I need to get to work on my garden.

Prayer
God, please help me today to continue learning how to live. Help me remain open-minded to new ideas so that I don't grow complacent. Amen

November 6

Thought for the day
Nothing we do, however virtuous, can be accomplished alone; therefore, we are saved by love.

Reinhold Niebuhr

Meditation
Although I have known my fair share of failures in life, I have also experienced success and triumph. It is a great feeling when one of my plans materializes into a worthwhile project and I achieve the rewards of my effort. It is wonderful to rise to the top of the heap...to have my fifteen minutes of fame. Being a person that has a core low self-worth, it is important for me to acknowledge when I have done well and reward myself with praise. But it is also important for me to recognize all the people who have helped me along the way. I owe all my successes today to the fine people I have met in the recovery circles of my community. People that are suffering or have suffered just as I did, people who have always been there for me when I was down. Without these folks in my life I do not know if I would still be alive. The genuine love and compassion that these people have shown me has become the inspiration I was lacking to be able to love myself...and today, it is through self-love that all things in my life are possible.

Prayer
God, help me remember how all the wonderful things in my life today have come about...by your grace and the loving, caring people that you have placed in my life. I thank you God for the many blessings that you have bestowed upon me. Amen

November 7

Thought for the day
Regret is an appalling waste of energy; you can't build on it;
it's only good for wallowing in.

Katherine Mansfield

Meditation
Depression has a funny way of getting all our regrets out for
amateur night in our brain. With the village idiot (our
depression's little messenger) seated in the front row, one by
one our regrets get up on the stage to entertain. Of course
the village idiot is delighted with the thickening woe and
despair that each ensuing act brings...so for an encore, he
suggests that all the regrets get on stage at once and begin
their solo performances simultaneously. As they begin to
bellow out their individual tragedies, the village idiot
scampers to the front of the stage to orchestrate the madness,
encouraging each regret to out-shout and out-perform the
other. Today, if you find yourself feeling regretful, just close
your eyes and imagine this scene playing out in your head.
When I do so I can't help but laugh...and laughter has a
funny way of getting our regrets off the stage, and making
the village idiot sit down for awhile.

Prayer
God, help me today to see how useless it is for me to waste
my energy wallowing in my regrets. Help me understand
that when I am filled with regretful thoughts, the only person
I am really thinking about is myself. Amen

November 8

Thought for the day
We have too many high sounding words, and too few actions
that correspond with them.

Abigail Adams

Meditation
Catecholamine neuro-transmitters, 3-ring chemical structure
/ Tricyclic antidepressants, Monoamine Oxidase (MAO)
Inhibitors, Serotonin reuptake inhibitors, melancholia,
neurasthenia, affective disorder, neurobiological disorder,
psychopharmacology...I have nothing but the utmost respect
for science and the medical community. If it were not for
their efforts, it could be argued that many of us would have
already perished. But I must never forget that it is not by
medication alone that my life has improved. I certainly have
to give an honorable mention to all the fine doctors and
therapists that I have encountered throughout my years of
struggling to find my way. But the human touch...when I
finally surrendered and allowed somebody to love me...if I
had to give up all but one thing relevant to my recovery
today, I'd let go of everything except the fellowship that I
have found. For without these wonderful people in my life, I
would truly be alone again.

Prayer
God, sometimes I can complicate the simplest and purest of
things in life. Help me today to continue in my spiritual
growth, and not force life along any faster than it is supposed
to be going. Amen

November 9

Thought for the day
Sometimes I wish life had a fast-forward button.

Dan Chopin

Meditation
Sometimes I wish my life did too. Sometimes I wish my life also had a mute button, reverse, hyperspace and channel buttons. Wouldn't that be great? Then whenever we found ourselves unhappy with our surroundings or circumstances, we could just change the channel. Or if somebody was chewing our ear off with some long story that we were totally disinterested in, we could hit the mute button and walk away until we had the time to hear the rest of the tale. When I am suffering from depression, all I want is the fast-forward button to help me escape the darkness. I used alcohol and drugs for years as my hyperspace button. If I was depressed, which was almost every day, I would hit hyperspace and disappear off the screen for a while. The problem with hyperspace is once I hit it; I had no control over where it would take me, or how long I would be gone. I also never knew where on the screen of life I would reappear. Sometimes the hospital sometimes jails, sometimes sleeping with my feet in my car and my body on the ground of a local bar parking lot...sometimes safely in my own bed. After years of that insanity, I just wanted to fast-forward to my death. Today I don't have the luxury of any of those buttons, but I do have a new and exciting button to use...the "courage to change my life" button. The neat thing about this button is that I can use it anytime that I wish.

Prayer
God, help me live my life in your speed not mine. Help me understand that I can change my life in any way that I desire if I am willing to make all the required sacrifices and efforts. Amen

November 10

Thought for the day
The closing years of life are like the end of a masquerade party, when the masks are dropped.

Arthur Schopenhauer

Meditation
Today, the idea of waiting to the closing years of my life to lose my masks and "get real" is appalling. I wore my masks, hiding behind them...lying, cheating, stealing, and hating myself for how phony I was...searching for myself...trying to determine which mask I really was. At the end, all that was left for me were the masks of comedy and tragedy...for I was a joke and my life was tragic. Today I can personify many different roles, yet I never have to stop being myself.

Prayer
God, I don't want to live my life behind the veil of masks. I want to continue to discover who I am and reveal that person to the world. Amen

November 11

Thought for the day
You only live once – but if you work it right, once is enough.
Joe E. Lewis

Meditation
One of my greatest fears is having my life pass me by and then discovering all the things that I wished I had done or said. Today my goal in life is not necessarily longevity, although I am currently not opposed to that proposition. My goal is to live life to its fullest potential. To have the courage and staying power to pursue all my hopes and dreams, and to settle with the understanding that what does not materialize in my life is directly related to a decision I made not to pursue it any longer. If I accept life on life's terms and work it right, then living once will naturally be enough.

Prayer
God, only you know when my physical life will end and my spirit will return to you. Let my life today be a proving ground for my spirit...let me remember how fragile, short, and precious my life truly is. Amen

November 12

Thought for the day
Life is a progress from want to want, not from enjoyment to enjoyment.

Samuel Johnson

Meditation
When we are in the grips of depression, we can know little enjoyment and much want. We often only want to "end it all", convinced that our opportunities to know true contentment have long since passed us by. Depression, leaving us deprived of happiness for perhaps years, has created within us an insatiable appetite for relief...relief which we conclude is available to us somewhere within the fulfillment of our want list. And so we get caught up in the illusion once again...the idea that some person, place, or thing can make us feel better. Today, our lives are no longer about living from want to want. Today we are learning by sharing our experience, strength and hope with each other, how to live from enjoyment to enjoyment.

Prayer
God, help me today not to settle for living from want to want. Help me learn how to live life from enjoyment to enjoyment and share my newfound joys with all that may benefit from them. Amen

November 13

Thought for the day
The good life, as I conceive it, is a happy life. I do not mean
that if you are good you will be happy – I mean that if you
are happy you will be good.

Bertrand Russell

Meditation
How happy are you today? If you cannot currently stake
your claim upon happiness, what obstacles are standing in
your way? Are you still allowing the old messages of self-
contempt to play as background music in your head? Are
you depressed and not treating it? We who have suffered
with depression know all too well the life of unhappiness.
We know how to try over and over again to feel happy, only
to have our best efforts wash out from beneath us leaving us
flat on our backs again. I do believe that a good life is a
happy life. I also know that for people like us, the pursuit of
happiness is not an easy one. We have to work a little harder
at it if we hope to obtain it. We have learned through our
shared experiences that together we stand a much better
chance of knowing the good life than we would standing
alone.

Prayer
God, my prayers go out to all my fellow depression sufferers
who are struggling today to know a simple happiness. Please
help us to continue to reach out to each other, to form
anonymous meetings in our communities, and be available
for on-line chats and phone conversations. Help us
remember that it is with each other, not by ourselves, that we
will find the happiness that we desire and deserve. Amen

November 14

Thought for the day
The difference between what we do and what we are capable
of doing would suffice to solve most of the world's
problems.

Gandhi

Meditation
My untreated depression had collapsed so heavily upon my
life that all of my confidence to succeed had been squeezed
completely out of me. After a few failed suicide attempts, I
sunk even lower into the murky waters of perceived
incompetence because, after all, I couldn't even take my own
life correctly. When I was younger, I was repeatedly told
that I had great potential if only I could find a way to smooth
out my way of living. As I proceeded to live my life, falling
short of all I could have been, I was constantly nagged by the
notion that I was such a huge disappointment and a waste of
human life. Today, in all fairness to myself, I understand
that I was not a bad person that needed to get good, I was a
sick person that needed to get well. By accepting this, I now
understand my true limitations and capabilities, and try each
day to live within the boundaries of both of them.

Prayer
God, please help me today to live within the boundaries of
my limitations and capabilities. Help me excel to my highest
potential, without setting myself up for failure by trying to
exceed my given limitations. Amen

November 15

Thought for the day
Sometimes, when one person is missing, the whole world seems depopulated.

Alphonse de Lamartine

Meditation
For years, that one person who was missing was I. I was emotionally unavailable to my family, unable to be an active participant in their lives because I wasn't able to be present in my own. My untreated depression had isolated me so much from the rest of the world that even when I was surrounded by my immediate family, I felt like an outsider who did not belong. Believing that my family would be happier without me, I would make myself physically unavailable by leaving the house for days on end. Alone on my bar stool, I would hammer down the drinks until I was so intoxicated that I would begin to believe that I really was important. It is ironic to me that alcohol and cocaine, the two substances that I was trying to kill myself with, probably kept me alive long enough to receive the professional help that I needed to treat my depression, alcoholism and chemical dependency. By doing so, I now am present in my life, clean and sober, and able to be an active participant in the lives of my family and friends.

Prayer
God, for years I was unavailable to so many people who loved me and wanted me in their lives. Help me today to share myself with others and be emotionally present in their lives. Amen

November 16

Thought for the day
'Mean to' don't pick no cotton.

Anonymous

Meditation
Sometimes, especially when we are suffering with a bout of depression, it is difficult to find the motivation to do the things we know we ought to be doing. We can get so caught up in the frivolous practice of trying to get out of it, that we actually expend more energy devising our escape from responsibility than would have been required to have just done it in the first place! It is important to my recovery that I maintain my commitments and do the things I say I'm going to do. When I am depressed, it is especially important that I force myself off the couch and into action. I don't have to accomplish everything everyday, but my actions are an outward sign of an inward desire to not allow depression to steal yet another day of my life away from me.

Prayer
God, when I am suffering from a bout of depression, help me get off the couch and into action. Help me acknowledge my efforts as an outward sign of my inward desire to not allow this illness to steal yet another day of my life from me. Amen

November 17

Thought for the day
People don't ever seem to realize that doing what's right is
no guarantee against misfortune.

William McFee

Meditation
It is wrong for me to expect that since I have been through
hell to get where I am today, I am now somehow shielded
from any future suffering. I have experienced many painful
emotions since I have begun my recovery process. What I
have found is that I am not shielded from life's problems, but
I am now empowered to successfully deal with its trials and
tribulations in a way that doesn't cause me any additional
harm. With the people in my life today, with the unity that
we so openly share with each other, I am certain I can endure
all things that my life may have to offer. We all are going to
experience misfortune...that's part of life. But if I am able
to successfully work through the adversity and find the
opportunities for spiritual growth that each misfortune
brings, then I will have learned how to truly live.

Prayer
God, please help me work through my misfortunes in life in
a way that will promote spiritual growth. Help me remember
that it has been through my painful past that I have turned to
you in prayer. Amen

November 18

Thought for the day
Without work all life goes rotten.

Albert Camus

Meditation
It has been estimated that depression has a cost impact on our economy in the amount of 43 billion dollars per year! Through lost production, medical costs, and lack of economic contributions by potential wage earners...nowhere is our economy able to operate without feeling the high tax that is directly related to this disease. The Beast: A Reckoning with Depression; Thompson. Many of us have lost jobs because of our depression, but it is unlikely that depression was listed as the cause of termination. Or maybe we just quit because we knew our employer was growing intolerant of our frequent absences. It is important that we be honest with ourselves regarding how this illness has affected our ability to function in the workplace. Think about how much money we have lost because of absenteeism alone. When we are in the bottom of the black hole, it is virtually impossible to perform even the simplest of tasks properly. So we have no choice but to miss yet another day of work. But today we have the responsibility to do our best to prevent ourselves from slipping that deep. We need to be ever alert for all the warning signs and to take action as soon as we suspect that a bout may be looming on the horizon.

Prayer
God, I have many financial responsibilities that I must meet everyday. Help me remember that by taking care of myself by treating my depression, I am able to meet my responsibilities and no longer place my financial burdens on others. By taking care of my responsibilities I also increase my sense of worth... to others as well as to myself. Amen

November 19

Thought for the day
When people make changes in their lives in a certain area, they may start by changing the way they talk about that subject, how they act about it, their attitude toward it, or an underlying decision concerning it.

Jean Illsley Clarke

Meditation
Change is difficult. Even when the necessity for change is obvious to everyone on the outside looking in...even when all the evidence suggests that the change will enhance the quality of our life, change often is easier said than done. Changing my attitude about depression was a big deal, but the change did begin to unfold once I made a decision to become open-minded to some new information regarding this disease. That was the first obstacle I had to overcome...a disease? Come on! I just had a lousy attitude, and once my life started to treat me right then my attitude would change into something a little more upbeat, right? By acceptance and making a decision to become open-minded to some new information, I was able to begin changing how I talked about depression, how I acted about it, and most importantly, I was able to change my attitude toward it.

Prayer
God, help me today to make the changes I need to make. Help me become open-minded to new information so that I may discover what needs changing in my life. Amen

November 20

Thought for the day
A single event can awaken within us a stranger totally
unknown to us. To live is to be slowly born.
Antoine de Saint-Exupery

Meditation
I was so afraid of the stranger who lived within me that I
tried repeatedly to kill both of us. I don't know of what I
was so afraid; he turned out to be one of the nicest guys I
know. It is amazing how I can look back on my life and
witness the landmarks that completely changed my direction.
Some of them are substantial, others barely noticeable. Yet
both impacted my life equally. Today I pay closer attention
to the "details", and worry less about the "big deals". I don't
take the homerun swing much any more...I'm looking for
the base hit. It is interesting to note that most big-league
homerun hitters often lead their teams in strikeouts. Today, I
enjoy the single events of my life and understand that life is
a process of perpetual rebirth.

Prayer
God, today help me slow down and enjoy the single events
of my life. Help me to be attracted to a life of perpetual
rebirth rather than looking for the big hit. Amen

November 21

Thought for the day
So lonely 'twas that God himself
Scarce seemed there to be.

Samuel Taylor Coleridge

Meditation
I should never soon forget the agony that was mine when I called out to God to save me from myself, only to find that my prayers would not take flight and leave my soul. So lonely was I when I believed that even my God found nothing worth salvaging from the wreckage of my life. So scarce were my hopes of ever feeling the zealousness for life that I had once known. How jealous was my heart of all the other people that God had chosen to love. I should never soon forget how God loved me when I could not love myself.

Prayer
God, often when I do not feel your presence in my life, my faith in your love for me wavers. Help me accept in my heart that your love for me is perfect and unconditional. Help me to remember that I should always turn to you for the guidance and inspiration that I so desperately need. Amen

November 22

Thought for the day
The tongue ever turns to the aching tooth.

Proverb

Meditation
When we are severely depressed, we can do little more than
turn all of our attention toward ourselves. We can become
extremely preoccupied with how worthless and hopeless we
are...how useless, ugly, lazy, selfish, boring, hypocritical,
judgmental, and dishonest we are. Stuck in our despair, we
have nothing left to give to the people in our lives who may
be depending on us...especially our children. They just
don't understand. We see the confusion, grief, and fear
within their eyes. They don't understand why we keep
pushing them away, why they can't seem to make us happy.
Feeling ashamed of ourselves, we become angry and start
finding fault with them, going to great lengths to prove that
if only these things were not occurring, then maybe we
wouldn't be so unhappy. In many ways untreated depression
destroys lives in the same way alcoholism does. I am so
grateful that I am finally seeing support groups forming
solely for the support of family members who have lived or
currently live with someone who suffers from this disease.

Prayer
God, depression not only takes its toll on us, but it also
adversely affects the lives of innocent children. Help us
recognize the negative impact this disease has on their lives
too. Amen

November 23

Thought for the day
Who will tell whether one happy moment of love or the joy
of breathing or walking on a bright morning and smelling the
fresh air, is not worth all the suffering and effort which life
implies...

Erich Fromm

Meditation
I have two sons who try my patience constantly. I have a
dog that does the same. My children will exhaust me with
their seeming inability to follow simple instructions and do
what they are told without being told to do it five times first.
My dog, well let's just say that I have been seriously
considering starting an Ala-dog meeting in my neighborhood
because he has obviously been damaged by my years of
drinking. Yet after a week of frustration, my oldest son will
bring home a 100% on a test, and the next morning, my
youngest will score a goal at the soccer game and I'll decide
once again that it is all worth it. I guess I can say the same
about living with depression. By the grace of God I got the
treatment that I needed. I often find myself becoming
extremely grateful that I am still alive to enjoy the special
moments in my life. Although it sometimes feels like long
hours and no fun, there is always that bright morning and
fresh air that occurs just when I need it the most.

Prayer
God, help me to always look forward to the rainbow after the
storm. Help me remember that my life is not always going
to be like a parade...that sometimes it is going to be painful
and feel only like work. Help me keep the faith that it will
all be worth it in the end. Amen

347

November 24

Thought for the day
Recovery is...overcoming the fear of living.
Anonymous

Meditation
I often am overtaken with anxious and fearful feelings for no apparent reason. I can become consumed with a sense of impending doom that seems to appear within me from nowhere. I have been troubled by these feelings for quite some time, and just recently began to discuss these unwelcome occurrences with my doctor. The neat thing about all of this is that I now have the tools to handle these situations in a healthy way. I no longer have to harm myself with alcohol, drugs, or suicidal thoughts. When I am fearful, it is important that I openly discuss my feelings with my support group and my doctor. It is such a relief to know that I don't have to go it alone. My recovery today is about overcoming my fears, not necessarily by ridding myself of them forever, but by being willing to address them, and then with the help of others, be free from them, one fear at a time.

Prayer
God, please help me to be free from my unwarranted fears today. Help me remember that I never have to be alone again...that I can always turn to the support I now have in my life. Amen

November 25

Thought for the day
There is no grief which time does not lessen and soften.

Edmund Spenser

Meditation
How do we overcome all the years that we were grief stricken by our untreated depression? How do we ever make amends to the people we had harmed during our darkest hour? We do it one day at a time. Today we try to live better than yesterday...we hold our tongue to prevent ourselves from say things that we might soon regret. We make a conscious effort to display a happy disposition...to become genuinely interested in the happenings of our family members' lives. We remember that each day that we are stepping in the right direction builds upon the previous day, and after a period of time, we have developed a history that is no longer painful to look upon, but rather one that we are happy to claim.

Prayer
God, today I want to live within the solution by no longer contributing to the problem. Help me walk and talk in a manner that is pleasing to you. Help me build a new history that I will be happy to claim. Amen

November 26

Thought for the day
Learning to trust is one of life's most difficult tasks.

Isaac Watts

Meditation
My life has been a long series of cliff climbing and cliff diving. I have exhausted myself many times as I struggled to keep my grip and swing my foot over the top of the mountain, only to let go at the last minute and plummet backward into the cold, dark waters below. Over the years, after being so close to the top only to fall back into the abyss, my intestinal fortitude had been shattered. I completely lost my will to try to climb the mountain, convinced that I knew what the outcome would be. I had completely lost all faith and trust in myself. Unable to believe in myself, I found it very difficult to trust others. I had become a pessimistic cynic who would scoff at even the simplest of truths, certain that they only could apply to the other guy. When I was near death I was faced with two choices...continuing my downward spiral with no evidence that I could stop my descent on my own, or trusting a foreign philosophy which asked me to let go and allow others to catch me before I fell to my catastrophic end. Today, I thank God I chose the latter.

Prayer
God thank you for teaching me how to trust again. At my lowest, I prayed to you for help and you answered my prayers by putting some wonderful people in my life who were willing to go to any length to help me if I would only let go and trust. Reluctantly, I did so...only because I saw no other way. I pray that you will help all my brothers and sisters who are currently struggling to trust, to just let go and allow the miracle to happen. Amen

November 27

Thought for the day
Humility is truth.
                    Erasmus

Meditation
Will you be rigorously honest with yourself today? If your friends or doctor ask you how things are going, will you say "great!" even though you know deep down inside that you aren't feeling all that good about yourself? It is easy to understand why we sometimes try to hide the truth about how we are feeling...it is a defensive measure that we use to keep ourselves from being harmed when we are most vulnerable. Yet by living our lives curled up tightly in a ball, we remain susceptible to many potential offenses while we deny ourselves all the opportunities that our lives may have in store for us. It is essential to my continual growth that I remain humble enough to be truthful about how I *really* am doing. It serves me no justice to pretend that I don't feel rotten when I am actually dying inside. I must remain willing to be rigorously honest about my feelings with the people in my life whom I can trust and count on to help me if need be.

Prayer
God, I pray for enough humility to be truthful with others and myself today. Help me remember that when I lie about how I am feeling, I am hurting myself by denying the opportunity for somebody to help me find my way. Amen

November 28

Thought for the day
I never think of the future. It comes soon enough.

Albert Einstein

Meditation
When I am suffering with a bout of depression, I usually feel very pessimistic about my life. I develop a "what difference does it make" attitude and begin to live very carelessly. When I think of the future, I often think about my funeral because I can no longer see much sense in living. Today I know to recognize these thoughts and feelings as symptoms of my illness and not the reality of my life. I understand that the only day I am entitled to live in is today...that yesterday is gone, and tomorrow never comes...that I need to be present in the moment of my life that is unfolding right now. When I am not wallowing in the past or fearing the future, I allow myself the benefit of all my faculties...and when I am 100% present in my life, I can successfully manage to negotiate my obstacles and take pleasure in the victories that I have achieved.

Prayer
God, help me today to live one day at a time. Help me to not wallow in the sorrow of the past, or be intimidated by the fear of the future, but to live within each moment of this day. Amen

November 29

Thought for the day
The aphorism, " As a man thinketh in his heart so is he", not only embraces the whole of a man's being, but is so comprehensive as to reach out to every condition and circumstance of his life. A man is literally what he thinks, his character being the complete sum of all his thoughts.

James Allen "As a Man Thinketh"

Meditation
If I accept this as a truth, which I do, then it is not difficult to understand how the disease of depression can destroy lives. Depression is a disease of our thoughts...a disease which attacks our self-worth on every front.   Left untreated, it weaves itself into the very fabric of our being until we eventually collapse beneath its relentless press.   Our heart succumbs,   and   we   literally   become   as   we thinketh...worthless, hopeless, pitiful, wastes of human life. Over the years, these diseased thoughts have forged our character into such disfigurement that we soon believe we are not even worthy of help...that we only deserve to die. Our punishment has been severe. But today we have begun the life long process of purging our hearts of the ill thoughts that depression has deposited in them...we have begun to learn that we are not worthless, but rather wonderful people who are worthy of recovery and love.

Prayer
God, help me continue to purge my heart of the impurities that depression has left behind. Help me use the many tools you have given me to prevent this illness from corrupting my character any more. Amen

November 30

Thought for the day
Obstacles are those frightful things you see when you take your eyes off your goal.

Henry Ford

Meditation
A few weeks after I started to treat my depression, I began to slowly lift out of the fog that I was in for over a year. I started to feel optimistic about my future again, and became very excited about all the opportunities that were awaiting me. But I also remember having a nagging fear that my new found freedom from the black hole would not last...that the bottom was going to fall out at any moment. I was afraid to feel good, afraid of falling from my high perch, afraid of how hard I would hit the ground if I did slip and fall. It took a few years for me to begin to really trust my recovery...to trust the doctors and therapists, to trust my recovering friends, to trust myself. But after experiencing numerous lapses into depression only to pull through quickly to the other side, I now have the confidence I lacked for so many years and a faith that reassures me that my obstacles are not walls, but doors for me to open.

Prayer
God thank you for the faith and confidence that has been bestowed upon me as a result of my recovery process. Thank you for the courage I now have to sct and achieve many of my goals. Amen

December 1

Thought for the day
Opportunity is missed by most people because it is dressed in overalls and looks like work.

Thomas Edison

Meditation
As a direct result of living with depression for so many years, many of us had grown accustomed to not starting much of anything because we were certain that it would fail. Others, myself included, were great starters, but horrible finishers. I was always concocting new recipes for feeling good about myself, and some of them did have merit. But I never seemed to have the staying power to see them through to their conclusion. Consequently, I spent a lot of time failing over the years, which in turn, only flamed the fires of my illness even more. I was always looking for the big hit...the instant gratification of the luck of the draw. I have since given up on the idea that good things will just happen. I am acutely aware of the labor that I must contribute to my life today...not only to gain materially...but spiritually as well.

Prayer
God, please protect me from the evils of complacency and laziness. Help me remember that what I hold most dear to my heart today, are the things that I had to work hard at to achieve. Amen

December 2

Thought for the day
Yesterday is history. Tomorrow is a mystery. And today?
Today is a gift. That's why we call it the present.

Babatunde Olatunji

Meditation
Living one day at a time is often easier said than done. With
all the things that we encounter in our daily living that
remind us of days gone by...and all the things that surround
and aspire us to set goals which we hope to achieve in the
future...staying within the present sometimes seems like a
idea that can only be fulfilled in fairy tales. Yet many of us
have found that if we wear the "one day at a time"
philosophy like a loose fitting garment, the benefits far
exceed the efforts we have to make to modify our way of
thinking about our lives. Of course we think about
tomorrow, and our memories are always present in our
minds, but today we understand that we do not have to *live* in
the past or the future. Today, we can practice keeping our
main focus on the here and now...not allowing our mind to
wander away from the gift we have been given...the present
moment.

Prayer
God, please help me today to rejoice in this present
moment...to be free from the regrets of the past and the fears
of the future. Amen

December 3

Thought for the day
The best things in life aren't things.
Art Buchwald

Meditation
At my lowest of lows, I would have traded everything I owned to be able to experience serenity and peace in my heart. All the *things* in my life had let me down. Even the magic I once had found in the bottle was gone. Nothing, absolutely nothing, was able to make me feel better...not sex, not drugs, not alcohol, not money, not prestige...nothing was able to fill the emptiness inside me. The only *thing* that has ever filled that awful void in my heart is love. First, the feeling of being loved by others unconditionally, then the feeling of self-love, and then, the assurance and comfort of the everlasting love of my Creator.

Prayer
God thank you for the unconditional love I have been shown by my friends, and the comfort of your everlasting love that I now know in my heart. God please help all those who are lost with this disease...to find the love and support that they so desperately need. Amen

December 4

Thought for the day
If a man is called a streetsweeper, he should sweep streets even as Michelangelo painted, or Beethoven composed music, or Shakespeare wrote poetry. He should sweep streets so well that all the hosts of heaven and earth will pause to say, Here lived a great streetsweeper who did his job well.

Martin Luther King, Jr.

Meditation
Today, I owe it to myself to be the best person I can possibly be regardless of what task awaits me. For years, unbeknownst to me, depression had been stifling my performance in all aspects of my life. Deep down inside, I always knew I could excel at whatever it was that I had to do...but for some reason I continually struggled to rise to the occasion and give it my best shot. Today I am determined to not allow this disease to deny me of the rewards that life has to offer. I'm not going to believe for one minute longer that I am worthless and undeserving of victories. I'm going to believe in my heart that if I do my best at even the simplest of chores...not settling for "good enough", but rather doing the absolute best that I can possibly do...then I also will hear the hosts in heaven saying, "here lived a great man who lived his life well".

Prayer
God, I settled for "good enough" too many times in my life. My untreated depression kept telling me not to even bother trying to succeed because I was worthless. Please help me to never believe the lies of this illness again. Help me identify and separate myself from the messages that depression sends, and quickly replace them with messages of positive reinforcement. Amen

December 5

Thought for the day
The best helping hand that you will ever receive is the one at the end of your own arm.

Fred Dehner

Meditation
No matter how persistently somebody tries to help us, if we are not willing to accept their help ...then obviously, all their unsolicited assistance will fall on deaf ears. Or if we are in complete denial as to whether we need help in the first place...then we will often become flat out rebellious to any suggestion that something may be wrong with us. But if we are the one who reaches out our hand...who picks up the telephone and calls for help, then we have placed ourselves in the position to make revolutionary changes in our entire attitude and outlook upon life. I am often reminded that my reprieve from depression is not magic or obtained through osmosis, it requires continual effort on my part. I have to remain willing to help myself...even when this illness is telling me otherwise.

Prayer
God help me continue to help myself by reaching out to those around me who are successfully treating their depression...one day at a time. Amen

December 6

Thought for the day
Many an opportunity is lost because a man is out looking for four-leaf clovers.

Unknown

Meditation
We all are familiar with the hopeful anticipation that is associated with wishful thinking. Even if the odds are against us, one million to one, we still cling to the possibility that good fortune may turn our way and we'll be the "one" this time. A great example of this is the state lottery. Nobody purchases a lottery ticket completely certain that they are going to lose, but the odds are grossly on the side of the state. For some of us, the pursuit of the four-leaf clover can become very detrimental to our health. We ignore the odds, and wager more time and money then we can afford to lose, in the hope that we will strike it rich. When we lose, we gamble more of our lives away in our effort to regain what has already been lost. Of course, for depression sufferers, this sort of thinking can be extremely dangerous because, with each new loss, we add fuel to our feelings of being a complete failure. Today I know in my heart that it is a much safer bet for me to practice prudence and reserve, rather than place my future in the roll of the dice.

Prayer
God, help me to be practical in my pursuit of happiness. Help me to not invest my time and money into ventures that will, based on the odds, probably leave me empty...in more ways than one. Amen

December 7

Thought for the day
If you don't know where you are going, you will probably
end up somewhere else.

Lawrence J. Peter

Meditation
Prior to being diagnosed with clinical depression, I often felt
completely lost in my life. I seemed to have thousands of
ideas and circumstances battling with each other in my brain
at all times, and I was never quite certain where I was going
to end up in this whirlwind of madness. After repeatedly
appearing in places that I didn't want to be...or in situations
that I found appalling, I soon became afraid to trust any of
my lonely thoughts. I realized that I had no evidence
whatsoever to support the notion that I was capable of
plotting a course of action for my life that would yield a
happy return. I became afraid to face each new day because
I seemed to have no control over my life. After years of
fighting off the terror, I finally buckled under this disease's
relentless pursuit and just let it run me over. And so it did.
Today, I no longer have to allow this illness or its related
symptoms to rule my life. I can start each day with a
hopefulness that I do understand where I am going...that I
can trust myself if I am treating my depression one day at a
time.

Prayer
God, please illuminate the path in which you want me to
walk. Show me the way to the truths in my life; protect me
from wandering astray. Amen

December 8

Thought for the day
If opportunity doesn't knock, build a door.

Milton Berle

Meditation
To me, one of the greatest tragedies that results from clinical depression, aside from suicide, is our loss of all willingness to create opportunity for ourselves. Depression stifles even the most talented of people from sharing their beauty and skills with the rest of the world because it convinces them that they are worthless and their efforts are substandard at best. We all lose when this illness, left untreated, denies us of the awesome brilliance of another human being living up to their fullest potential. To me, that is very sad indeed.

Prayer
God, if we don't hear opportunity knocking, please help us all regain our complete willingness to build a door. Help us today to be the best we can be no matter what it is that we do. Help us always encourage each other to give life our best effort. Amen

December 9

Thought for the day
Only those who will risk going too far can possibly find out
how far one can go.

T.S. Eliot

Meditation
I have not suffered through suicide attempts, the "cold
sweats" and shakes at numerous "detox" centers, and
perhaps hundreds of hours of painful psychotherapy, to not
take advantage of all that my life has to offer. I've been
down long enough. Today, by the grace of God, I believe I
can do anything I choose to do if I am willing to do the
legwork. My God can move mountains...but I'm often
asked to bring the shovel. I don't believe it is advantageous
for me to take foolish risks in my life, but I do realize that
there are some healthy risks which are necessary and well
worth considering. Usually, it is simply a matter of stepping
out of my comfort zone and trying something new. Today,
as a result of treating my depression and living one day at a
time, I have the willingness to take healthy risks, and the
faith that God did not save me from drowning just to smash
me against the rocks of the shore.

Prayer
God thank you for the many opportunities I am blessed with.
Thank you for the willingness I now have to take healthy
risks, and the faith that you will see me through to the
rightful conclusion of my physical life. Amen

December 10

Thought for the day
Even if you're on the right track, you'll get run over if you just sit there.

Will Rogers

Meditation
I'm great for getting on the right track. After a setback in my life, I have repeatedly been able to pick up the pieces of my shattered dreams, quickly duct tape them back together, and then jump right back onto the next "right track" that presents itself in my life. The problem I have always encountered has been my ability to sustain my *loco*-motion for any considerable length of time. I have always seemed to run out of steam, usually in the middle of a busy intersection. Today I am certain my untreated depression had much to do with my inability to maintain my motion in life. I now realize and accept that if I neglect to monitor and treat this disease, it will continually derail my hopes and dreams, and possibly kill me.

Prayer
God, please help me today to maintain my motion on the track of recovery. Help me continually monitor my engine for symptoms of depression, and maintain the preventive maintenance schedule that has been prescribed for me. Amen

December 11

Thought for the day
When nothing seems to help, I go look at a stonecutter hammering away at a rock perhaps a hundred times without as much as a crack showing in it. Yet at the hundredth blow it will split in two, and I know it was not that blow that did it but all that had gone before.   **Jacob Riis**

Meditation
After reading this quotation for the first time, I was inspired by the wisdom and perseverance that the stonecutter seemed to possess. He learned from experience the results he could expect if he kept hammering away at the rock. The thought of quitting probably never entered his mind because he had grown familiar with the process at hand. But after a second read, I discovered what I consider a peculiar twist to this quote. The first few words..."When nothing seems to help..." reminds me of how I will so frequently exhaust myself in search of the answer to "why" by looking in all the wrong places, instead of drawing upon my own experiences and recollections to find the wisdom I am seeking. Often, we trouble ourselves greatly by pursuing answers to our life that we already know. We sometimes complicate even the simplest of tasks by scrambling around frantically in search of the correct course of action when, if we just slow down for a moment and regain our composure, the peaceful solution, based on our past experiences, will come to us.

Prayer
God, help me today to maintain the perseverance that I need to see the circumstances of my life through to their conclusion. Help me relax when crisis enters my life...to consider whether I have any past experiences that may better help me deal with the situation I am presently encountering. Amen

December 12

Thought for the day
Our greatest glory is not in never failing, but in rising up every time we fail.

Ralph Waldo Emerson

Meditation
For many of us who treat depression with anti-depressants, the feelings of failure which we often encounter when a certain type of medication doesn't work for us, or has side effects that we cannot bear, is depressing all in itself. I went through a two-year period when the medication I was taking would only be effective for three to four months, and then the bottom would fall out again. I remember how frustrated and sometimes embarrassed I was to have to call my doctor and tell her that I was in trouble again. Before I truly accepted depression as an illness, every time the medication that I was on failed to help, I would conclude that somehow I had failed...like there was something I was doing wrong. Today I accept that I am going to experience failures in my life. I understand that when I'm treating my depression with anti-depressants, I might go through a series of medications before I find the one that helps me. I understand that the most important thing I can do for myself today is to not let these minor setbacks be translated as failures in my brain, and to always get back up every time I slip and fall.

Prayer
God, please grant me the courage to pick myself up when I am down. Help me understand that some of my setbacks are actually teaching me a valuable lesson and should not be translated into the notion that I am a failure. Amen

December 13

Thought for the day
Someday is not a day of the week.

Unknown

Meditation
How often is it that we say to ourselves, " If I don't feel any
better tomorrow, then I'll call the doctor"? Or, " I don't
think I'm depressed, I just have a lot of stressful things
happening in my life right now, and after things get back to
normal, I'll feel better". Many of us are guilty of scheduling
all of our happiness on Someday, February 30th. We work
and we plan, we manipulate and control, we suffer
needlessly by letting our depression go unchecked, and
before we realize it...someday never comes and we have lost
our opportunity to do those great things which we once
dreamed of. Today is our Someday that we once only hoped
for. Right here, right now, we have every right to enjoy our
life. Take care of yourself today by doing something special
for yourself. Go have some ice cream with a friend. Buy
yourself a new book or participate in a long lost hobby. But
whatever you do...don't let today pass you by without
having one good laugh and a little bit of fun.

Prayer
God, help me not put off having fun today. Often I get
myself so wrapped up in the seriousness of life that I fail to
see the humor in it. Help me to practice relaxation and to
enjoy the softer moments that my life has to offer. Amen

December 14

Thought for the day
Remember that a kick in the ass is a step forward.

Unknown

Meditation
I no longer have an excuse to wallow in the sadness that is brought on by a bout with depression. I do not have the right to neglect myself...causing all those that come in contact with me to be exposed to my suicidal disposition. I have friends in my life today who will not participate in any of my pity parties. They will not accept my leaving depression unchecked...they will give me a kick in the ass when I'm having a little trouble finding the motivation that is required for me to take care of myself. Although it may not feel like it at the time, I am truly blessed to have people in my life today who will not enable me in my sickness, but will be stern with me when I am wavering in my recovery.

Prayer
God, every once in a while, I need a good old fashioned kick in the ass to get myself back onto the right track. I thank you for the people in my life today who are not afraid to administer the proper motivation that I need from time to time...I think they call it tough love. Amen

December 15

Thought for the day
When the horse is dead, get off.

Unknown

Meditation
When I consider how many times I have returned to a contaminated well to draw upon its water, each time convinced that "this time it would be different"...only to pull up an old pail of sour, sickening drink. And then to ignore the obvious and gulp from the ladle as if the water looked like it just bubbled out of a sparkling, fresh mountain spring...it embarrasses me to consider how arrogant and foolish I must have appeared. I also can envision myself sitting on a dead horse, kicking its bloated sides, with the absolute certainty that it is sure to rise and gallop again. I thank God that I no longer have to live like that.

Prayer
God, help me to remain humble enough to notice if my "horse" is dead. Amen

December 16

Thought for the day
Failure doesn't mean you are a failure…it just means you haven't succeeded yet.

Robert Schuller

Meditation
I often find it difficult to prevent these signals from getting crossed. I can very easily internalize an outward failure as evidence that I'm a failure. Today I understand that low self-esteem is always at the root of any self-condemnation, and that depression plays a major role in my feelings of worthlessness. One of the key components to my successful treatment of this disease is to restore my self-esteem to what is considered a healthy level. To do so, I have to look at the evidence of my life through sober eyes. Each day that I don't hold another person responsible for how I feel or harbor any suicidal thoughts, I have succeeded. Each day that I make myself available to another human being that is in trouble and really needs somebody to lean on, I have successfully discovered the meaning of my life. I am learning that these are the things that really define my success today, and that the rest of the "stuff"…it never really mattered.

Prayer
God, please help me today not to internalize any of my outward failures. Help me to remember that by taking care of myself and helping others, I am succeeding everyday.
Amen

December 17

Thought for the day
The greatest oak was once a little nut who held its ground.

Unknown

Meditation
We all were little nuts at one time and we all have been a little nuts many times since. For many of us who have suffered from acute clinical depression, the feeling that we were completely losing our minds is very familiar. Our attempts to attach rational thinking onto our irrational behaviors had failed. The people that we were blaming for our despair were acquitted by what little common sense we had left in our minds, and so all that we were left with was ourselves...and we quickly convicted ourselves as worthless wastes and sentenced ourselves to death. By the grace of God we have remained...we have held our ground long enough to get help and to be restored to sanity. But many do not make it. Each year, an estimated 30,000 Americans get washed away in a flashflood of depression. Left to their own devices, they no longer held the strength to hold own. Had we been in their lives, we could have fortified their resolve...we could have helped them make it through another day.

Prayer
God, it grieves me to consider how many people are alone and suffering needlessly with this disease called depression. Please help them. Amen

December 18

Thought for the day
When I was a Boy Scout, we played a game when new Scouts joined the troop. We lined up chairs in a pattern, creating an obstacle course through which the new Scouts, blindfolded, were supposed to maneuver. The Scoutmaster gave them a few moments to study the pattern before our adventure began. But as soon as the victims were blindfolded, the rest of us quietly removed the chairs. I think life is like this game. Perhaps we spend our lives avoiding obstacles we have created for ourselves and in reality exist only in our minds. We're afraid to apply for that job, take violin lessons, learn a foreign language, call an old friend, write our Congressman – whatever it is that we would really like to do but don't because of personal obstacles. Don't avoid any chairs until you run smack into one. And if you do, at least you'll have a place to sit down.

Pierce Vincent Eckhart

Meditation
I liken the symptoms of depression to this game. When I am lost in the black hole, the darkness serves as the blindfold and my despair creates an obstacle course that really only exists in my mind. But unlike this innocent game, left untreated, my depression attaches shackles to my feet and handcuffs me behind my back. Then it sends me out to negotiate life. It places me in the middle of a superhighway at rush hour and tells me that there is really no point in struggling to save myself. It tells me that my obstacles are too great in number...that I might as well just jump in front of the next vehicle to get the inevitable over with as soon as possible. It continually bombards me with lies about my surroundings and...once the blindfold is lifted, I find myself back at home comfortably seated in my favorite chair.

372

Prayer

God, help me remember that when I am suffering with a bout of depression I cannot trust all that I am thinking and feeling. Help me remember that once I pull through, I will be able to look back and see that things were not as bad as I thought. Amen

December 19

Thought for the day
If it isn't broken, let's take it apart and see why not.

Unknown

Meditation
I have made a career out of paralysis by analysis...the fine art of complicating even the simplest of things to the point that nothing gets done. Motivated by the fear of the next bad thing that could happen in my life to cause me to spiral uncontrollably into the dark depths of depression, I had become vigilantly guarded against feeling good. If anything in my life started to feel comfortable or enjoyable, I would dissect it beyond recognition. I had reached a point in my life that I trusted absolutely nobody because of how badly they could hurt me, and I had zero tolerance for myself because I felt like such a freakish failure. Today I know to leave well enough alone. I am learning how to trust the recovery process and the people that are part of it. More importantly, I am discovering that I can count on myself to do "the next right thing" whenever I feel as if I am beginning to slip away.

Prayer
God, help me always to nurture my faith in you and your divine plan for me. Help me continue to trust my recovery process and the wonderful people that are part of it. Amen

December 20

Thought for the day
Waste your money and you're only out of money, but waste
your time and you've lost a part of your life.

Michael Leboeuf

Meditation
Every second of every minute, every minute of every hour,
every hour of every day...no matter how much effort we
have made to disrupt its cadence, time, never missing a step,
marches on. For most of my life, I have felt as though I were
merely a spectator to the parade of the "times of my life".
How I wished that I could have been part of it, but my
depression, undiagnosed and therefore untreated, kept me
from believing that I had any right to participate in the
happenings of my life. Today I know that if I'm waiting for
a special invitation to join in on the procession, I am going to
be sadly disappointed. I have to jump out and join in...and
then, with the support of others, learn how to lead my own
parade.

Prayer
God, help me today not to surrender my precious life to
depressed thinking. Help me to jump out and join into the
parade that is my life. Amen

December 21

Thought for the day
Hurt people, hurt people.
Anonymous

Meditation
There have been times in my life when, in a fit of rage, I
have hurt people badly. There have also been times when I
was suffering severely from depression, that I afflicted others
harshly with word and deed. I have also been on the
receiving end of another hurt person's thoughts and actions.
Today I make no excuses for either party; I just understand it
as a sad truth. Hurt people, hurt people.

Prayer
God, there are so many hurt people hurting each other in this
world today. Help me remember that although I may not be
able to change them, I am now able to change myself...to
stop hurting and to stop hurting others. Amen

December 22

Thought for the day
I give myself, sometimes, admirable advice, but I am
incapable of taking it.

Mary Wortley Montagu

Meditation
At times, the distance between advice and action can seem
endless. I often times will find myself offering up some
wonderful words of wisdom to somebody who may have
asked me for my opinion, only to realize in the middle of my
dissertation, that if I were to apply only half of what I was
saying to my own life, I would be a much better person for it.
Today I pay closer attention to what I am saying to others. I
try to practice what I preach, so to speak. I have learned that
talk is cheap. If I'm offering advice that I am not adhering to
myself, I feel like a hypocrite and a liar. And feeling this
way is cancerous to the spiritual condition which I have
worked so hard to obtain.

Prayer
God, please help me today to maintain a level of honesty that
convicts me to practice what I preach. Help me remember
that what I have always found most attractive in others was
not their words, but rather their deeds. Amen

December 23

Thought for the day
At bottom every man knows well enough that he is a unique human being, only once on this earth; and by no extraordinary chance will such a marvelously picturesque piece of diversity in unity as he is, ever be put together a second time.

Nietzche

Meditation
How often do you feel like a "marvelously picturesque piece of diversity"? I can say with complete certainty that I have never felt that good about myself. But, as a result of the continual efforts that I am making on a daily basis to restore my depression-ravaged self-esteem to that of holding myself in somewhat of high regard, I don't rule out the possibility that someday I could feel that grandly about myself. I believe most people don't realize how truly precious they are...even the folks who already appear to be completely full of themselves. When I consider this quotation on a spiritual level rather than on a superficial humanistic level, I can begin to understand how unique and unrepeatable my life truly is.

Prayer
God, help me today to understand how unrepeatable and unique my life truly is. Help me continue to repair my depression-ravaged self-esteem so that I may feel like a "marvelously picturesque piece of diversity". Amen

December 24

Thought for the day
'Tis peace of mind, lad, we must find.

Theocritus

Meditation
My mind, with the restlessness of a two-year old child and the stability of an infant's first steps...my mind has often left me breathless in my pursuit to contain it. Chasing it around, trying to clean up all of its messes, never quite catching up with it, staying up all night trying to rock it to sleep; in the past my mind has not allowed me much peace. All that I ever really desired, all that I was ever pursuing, was peace of mind and serenity in my heart. But my unruly mind, stubborn beyond its years, has always kicked and screamed...throwing embarrassing temper tantrums when it wasn't getting its own way. Lacking the parenting skills I needed, I would always succumb to my wayward thinking and let it set about on a dangerous course of action that could have possibly killed me. After years of battling with this child, I finally surrendered to the idea that if I loved this "little hell-raiser" I would seek some professional guidance. That decision has saved both of our lives.

Prayer
God, help me today to know peace of mind and serenity of the heart. When my life seems to be getting unruly, help me remember that I can always call for help. Amen

December 25

Thought for the day
Because I have been athirst
I will dig a well that others may drink.
Arabian proverb

Meditation
With an estimated 20 million Americans suffering from depression at any given moment, and 340 million people world-wide suffering from some variation of a mood disorder, it is easy to see that there are many who are still "athirst" for relief from their parched lives. We who have experienced the moment of clarity, who have accepted depression as a treatable medical condition rather than a sin, have been given a "well of life" from which we now live. We have so much to offer those who are still lost in the darkness of the black hole...some who will die alone today. The greatest responsibility that we have today is to help each other live with this illness so that none of us have to die from it.

Prayer
God, I have been blessed with the awareness and the acceptance that I suffer from a disease called depression, and that there are many successful ways to treat it. Help me now to carry this wonderful message of hope to all that may still be suffering. Amen

December 26

Thought for the day
I am not bound to win, but I am bound to be true. I am not bound to succeed, but I am bound to live up to what light I have.

Abraham Lincoln

Meditation
This quotation reminds me of the song..."This little light of mine, I'm gonna let it shine..." As silly as I think it is on an intellectual level, spiritually it gives me the warm "fuzzies". The recognition of a "little light of mine" that is capable of shining and perhaps radiating warmth into somebody else's life...we all have a light that we are bound to live up to. When we are depressed, it feels as though that light has been extinguished, but it burns on. As long as our heart beats, that little light burns on. Let your light shine today. Do something for someone special. Refuse to let depression shade your wonderful illumination. Feel the warmth that is deep down inside of you...smile awhile in the mirror. Make the stupidest faces you can make until you laugh at yourself, then go to work remembering how silly life really is. Oh, and by the way, if you are familiar with the song, you won't be able to get it out of your mind for awhile. You're welcome.

Prayer
God, please help me not to clutter my life up so much that I block the illumination of my "little light inside". Help me today to let it shine, let it shine. Amen

December 27

Thought for the day
Rescue me from the mire, do not let me sink, deliver me
from those who hate me, from the deep waters. Do not let
the floodwaters engulf me or the depths swallow me up or
the pit close its mouth over me.

Psalm 69:14-15 NIV

Meditation
Pretty strong language. Perhaps the author was over-
exaggerating his despair somewhat. Maybe not. To a person
who has never felt as though they were going to be
swallowed by the depths, these words may be little more
than literary hyperbole. Similarly, there may be a lack of
understanding when we relate our feelings (or complete lack
of feeling) to a person who has never suffered from
depression. Many people confuse feeling depressed...a
normal human experience...with depression, which is
outside the range of normal human experience. So to some,
this psalmist's words may be overstated. And our feelings
may seem overstated as well when we attempt to verbalize
them. But that doesn't mean that they're not authentic.
Those who haven't experienced deep depression may not
understand; may even make us question the validity of our
feelings. As one who has been there, I validate your
feelings. As for the floodwaters or the depths or the pit, they
can be overcome. We need not let them consume us. There
is healing and recovery and an end to those feelings. And I
say these things as one who has been there too.

Prayer
Lord, you are my rope when I am sinking. You are my
lifeline when I'm drowning. No matter how deep the depths
are that threaten to swallow me, I know that you are greater

still. It is at these times that I need you to lift me up, because alone, I have no choice but to succumb. Thank you for your love and for carrying me when I cannot go on alone. Amen

December 28

Thought for the day
Take away love and our earth is a tomb.
Robert Browning

Meditation
When we were suffering from depression, it robbed us of all feelings of love because we felt completely unlovable. Consequently, it was difficult for us to love anything or anybody else because we had no love for ourselves. Isolated, we felt completely separated from the rest of the world. We were certain that nobody felt the way that we did...that we were locked into a torturous hell that was designed by God to punish us for being the worthless, "no good" person that we were certain we had become. Our earth was our tomb, and living within it no longer made sense...we were convinced that we really should be dead. Today I recognize feelings of being unlovable as a symptom of this disease. I no longer accept the feeling as factual...as quickly as I possibly can, I challenge it by examining the evidence that it claims to have against me, and soon I discover that it is once again trying to bear false witness regarding who I really am.

Prayer
God, please help me today to remember how empty life is when I lose my capacity to love. Help me to not allow the feelings of depression to once again convict me as unlovable. Amen

December 29

Thought for the day
In thy face I see the map of honor, truth, and loyalty.
William Shakespeare

Meditation
The camaraderie I have felt and the fellowship I have found since I was first diagnosed with clinical depression has been more rewarding than I could have ever anticipated. For within the fellowship I have found, in the faces of my peers, the pain of experiencing the exact same hell that I have been through and the hope that I may also know a life of happiness, joy, and freedom if I am willing to follow their path.

Prayer
God, please help me today not to take the wonderful fellowship that I have been blessed with for granted. Help me remember that if I am to expect this support to always be available to me, I must always remain available to it. Amen

December 30

Thought for the day
To live well is nothing else but to love God.

St. Augustine

Meditation
My faith today is that a Divine Creator does exist. I believe that there is a Great Spirit that dwells in all things at all times...a Spirit of God's everlasting love and compassion that may only be felt when my mind, heart and soul enter into accord with this Spirit. If I am fostering hate and discontent within me, I will know only a rage-ridden life. But, if I am prayerfully cultivating spirits of goodwill, then I may be considered "living well" to know the love of God. If I am taking care of myself, treating my depression one day at a time, then I am loving myself...and to love myself is to love my God.

Prayer
God, I pray for the willingness to continue on my journey of spiritual renewal. Help me remember that by taking care of myself I am demonstrating self-love. Amen

December 31

Thought for the day
The influence of a beautiful, helpful, hopeful character is contagious, and may revolutionize a whole town.

Eleanor H. Porter

Meditation
After a failed suicide attempt, some of us have had to deal with the embarrassment of seeing our neighbors after we have been released from the hospital. Its hard to keep this sort of thing a secret...the sirens, police and paramedics always seem to bring out the neighbors. And there we are, out cold again. Either an overdose or dangerously drunk, perhaps with lacerations on our arms and neck...people can't help but to talk about us. They have no idea what we are going through and they probably never will. I have family members who will always consider me a "messed up person" who can never be trusted. After years of abstinence from alcohol and drugs, treating my depression one day at a time, they refuse to let me out of their distorted, misinformed perceptions. The truth is...they don't even know me anymore. It is sad that we have to deal with this shame and other people's scorn, but unfortunately it is best for us to just accept it and move on. Today I don't let anybody hold me down. I do what I can each day to help somebody who is hurting. All that I can hope for is that my efforts may influence some person's life in a positive way.

Prayer
God, please help me to grow into a beautiful, helpful, hopeful character...with a contagious spirit that may influence another person's life in some positive way. Amen

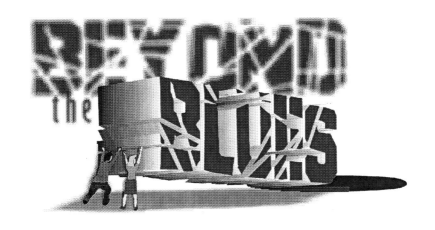

Treating Depression One Day at a Time

Index

A
Acceptance...9, 24, 68, 75, 211, 214, 224, 235, 245, 306
All or nothing thinking...40, 67, 186, 317
Ambitions...40, 229, 239, 250, 358
Anger...162, 376
Anti-depressants...86, 107, 248, 286, 327, 332, 366
Asking for help...8, 90, 92, 138, 379

B
Black hole...74, 84, 92, 123, 239, 380
Blaming others...75, 97, 99, 101, 121, 137, 371

C
Change...40, 153, 168, 201, 260, 264, 285, 297, 308, 343
Complacency...328, 329, 355
Contemplating death...94, 97, 100, 108, 141, 185
Courage...31, 128, 178, 244, 333

D
Dealing with life...32, 227, 365
Denial...161, 236, 334
Depressed thoughts...42, 233, 353
Depression as an illness...17, 29, 37, 133, 194, 212, 259
Depression left untreated...108, 115, 139, 161, 185, 204, 288
Describing depression...10, 163, 182, 346
Deserving recovery...18, 62, 113, 114, 143, 161

E
Expectations...41, 48, 105
External conditions...36, 43, 97, 99

F
Faith...57, 101, 134, 144, 160, 145, 307
Fear of failure...220, 252, 324, 354, 355, 370
Fear...26, 106, 118, 119, 166, 184, 318, 319, 348
Feeling phony...115, 122, 334, 377
Fellowship...11, 23, 30, 122, 145, 202, 253, 272, 332, 385
Forgiveness...268, 270

G
God...50, 57, 62, 69, 72, 98, 105, 160, 164, 188, 192, 216, 254, 311, 312, 345, 386
Gratitude...13, 25, 95, 96, 102, 234, 325, 326
Growth...30, 167, 180, 293, 294
Guilt...24, 31

H
Happiness...53, 91, 116, 181, 336, 367
Hate...191, 319
Helping others...79, 93, 102, 109, 129, 231, 251, 261, 371
Honesty...58, 171, 271
Hopes and dreams...16, 23, 34, 39, 41, 62, 81, 118, 222, 260, 335, 360, 364
Humility...35, 45, 38, 351

I
Identifying feelings...155, 162, 220, 235, 256, 280, 308, 309, 334, 384
Insane thinking...66, 90, 189, 206, 249, 295, 296, 320, 361, 369
Isolation...94, 169, 200, 257, 267

J
Judging others...213, 241, 276, 293, 299

K
Keeping it simple...33, 37, 69, 76, 130, 219, 261, 300, 310

L

Limitations...60, 67, 90, 269, 338
Living in the moment...104, 264, 352
Living in the past...223, 274, 296
Living one day at a time...68, 117, 262, 304, 349, 356
Living with depression...20, 33, 77, 85, 136, 164, 177, 237, 246, 273, 347, 372, 387
Loneliness...55, 141, 146, 287
Lost opportunity...28, 51, 199, 290, 362
Love...56, 85, 192
Lowest points...45, 52, 89, 112, 188, 211, 357

M

Making comparisons...61, 111, 206, 232
Measuring success... 330, 360
Miracles...93, 100, 147, 211, 302, 311, 321

O

Opportunities...11, 73, 282, 354

P

Patience...65, 96, 103, 107, 117, 242, 315, 347
Patterns of behavior...114, 174
Peace...35, 47, 54, 193, 316
Perseverance...65, 70, 77, 124, 134, 147, 186, 205, 350, 363
Powerlessness...321
Prayer...69, 83, 208, 263, 283

R

Recovery...21, 55, 120, 131, 148, 178, 339, 348, 368, 382
Regret...331
Renewal...91, 98, 103, 327, 344
Resentment...213, 258
Responsibility...59, 66, 140, 247, 277, 342

S

Seeking knowledge...22
Self-analysis...56, 63, 126, 166, 198, 203, 221, 313, 374
Self-esteem...88, 95, 152, 252, 303, 315, 378
Self-love...29, 46, 56, 78, 80, 85, 150, 173, 240, 270, 291
Self-medicating...18, 28, 36, 82, 139
Self-worth...153
Sense of urgency...12, 19
Separating from the illness...243
Solitude...143, 159, 176
Spiritual bankruptcy...156, 172, 323
Spiritual growth...43, 50, 87, 218, 289, 301, 341
Suffering...71, 119, 128, 159, 190, 275, 314
Suicide...44, 126, 191, 266
Surrendering...51, 292, 322

T

Taking action...15, 16, 72, 79, 111, 118, 154, 224, 306, 340, 355, 375
Treating depression...7, 14, 38, 64, 86, 174, 210, 228, 261, 265, 305, 326, 359, 381

U

Unity in recovery...27, 34, 110, 140, 195, 278, 325, 337

W

Warning signs...187, 209, 216, 217, 230, 238, 255, 298
Willingness...134, 150, 171, 197, 215, 237, 257, 279, 281, 284, 359
Worry...49, 193

Share it with a friend....

To order additional copies of Beyond the Blues, please send a check or money order in the amount of $18.95 plus $3.95 shipping and handling to:

Beyond the Blues
2411 Filbert Ave.
Mt. Penn, PA 19606

Please rush me:
_____ Copies of Beyond the Blues – Treating Depression One Day at a Time

My check is enclosed for $_____.

Name_____

Address_____

City_____ State_____
Zip_____